ENDORSEMENTS

It is a true gift when one of our fellow earth travelers allows us to see so deeply into their li Its sacred. Phoebe na gives us that gift with grea and wisdom. We get to follow h er powerful journey and it become ng a thread of golden light on the p becoming oneself. A beautiful invitation to allow everything we feel, we experience, to find its place within us.

-Gisela Stromeyer, Healer, Teacher
and Author of *Just Like That:
Poems, Paintings And Practices*

I love the book. Love everything about it. The stories shared (it takes guts to share like that) are not only fascinating, but they definitely open doors for contemplation. More than once, I paused to reflect on things in my own experience. Phoebe leads people through a journey with distinct challenges at each stage. The questions at each part remind me of stopping along the road to pause at a rest stop with a great view. Pause and do some work... but work that feels guided and supported.

-Jeanmarie Paolillo, Teacher and
Author of *The Vibe-A-Thon:
Creating Your Life From The Inside Out*

Phoebe is profoundly, wholeheartedly, dedicated to the path of healing. Every time I am in her presence, she shows up fully to share her whole self—with honesty, creativity, and vulnerability. Her teaching and writing is deeply rooted in her lived experience.

-Jillian Pransky, Teacher and
Author of *Deep Listening*

Dear Radiant One...

An Emotional Recovery Story and Transformational Guide to Embody the Dance of Life

PHOEBE LEONA

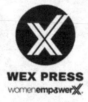

WEX PRESS
womenempøwerX.

An Imprint for GracePoint Publishing (www.GracePointPublishing.com)

GracePoint Matrix, LLC
624 S. Cascade Ave
Suite 201
Colorado Springs, CO 80903
www.GracePointMatrix.com
Email: Admin@GracePointMatrix.com
SAN # 991-6032

A Library of Congress Control Number has been requested and is pending.

ISBN: (Paperback) 978-1-955272-17-9
eISBN: 978-1-955272-18-6

Books may be purchased for educational, business, or sales promotional use.
For bulk order requests and price schedule contact:
Orders@GracePointPublishing.com

Thanks for buying *Dear Radiant One*! You can access more content—photos, poems, and videos—directly from Phoebe Leona designed to accompany the book and enrich your experience.

Open the camera app on your smart phone, direct it at this image, and you will automatically be redirected to the embedded link through your web browser.

In MEMORY of Dad, so you don't forget.

And Gabby, this is the sound of my soul.

Table of Contents

ACT TWO: DARK DANCES OF THE SOUL

ACT THREE: GRAND JETE INTO THE SUN

FINALE

Letter to Radiant One

Dear Radiant One,

This book is meant for you, and I am grateful you answered the call to hold it in your hands and page through to see what is here for you now.

This book has gone through a few transformations, just like we all do. It's gone through a couple of different titles and formats but the intention to share my story for you has been the same the entire time: to share the radiance of truth. Maybe others who know and have been part of this journey will have other perspectives, and so they should—that's their truth and theirs to honor fully. But this story I am choosing to share is my authentic story, one that no one has heard before.

The original title, Variably Cloudy with Abundant Sunshine, came to me on a day I will never forget. I woke up after two months of grieving my father's death, a relationship you will soon learn was rather complicated. I felt the warm spring sunlight shine on my face as my eyes began to open, and I took a breath that felt like a breath of fresh hope. I looked at my phone and saw the forecast, "Abundant Sunshine" and it felt like the long, dark, winter of grief was finally lifting. A few hours later, I found out that my fifteen-year marriage was coming to an end, and clouds rolled back in. The title came to me the next morning when I was taking a shower. I didn't know what was ahead for me, but I knew I had a choice to let the clouds take over my light or continue to hold onto my light and shine out abundantly despite what the weather did to cover me up. It's been a long eight-year journey since that day; a journey of self-discovery and emotional recovery that tested my radiance in many ways. But as I sit here now with the bright blue skies overhead, a cool breeze, and a warm sun beaming on me, I know I did it. I am still making the choice every day to embody my radiance.

This is where you come in, dear one, and truly, you have been here this whole time, living your own life, making your own choices, some days brighter, others gloomier; it's all good. You are here now.

Think of this as my love letter to you. For those gloomier days, I share with you my shadows of chaos, anxiety, fear, anger, resentment, grief, numbness, sadness, shame, guilt, and the practices that helped me express, regulate, or transform them into something else. My hope for you is they resonate, meet you where you are, and help you move beyond. Through my relationships with joy, gratitude, confidence, connection, love, peace, serenity, inspiration, trust, and patience, I share my love letters to these emotions and the practices that helped me so you can invite more of those emotions into your life and celebrate your lightness of being.

If you picked up this book, trust that you need this; we all need this right now. As I write for you in 2021, a great shift is occurring, and whenever you read this, it probably is still happening on some level within you. Think of this as an invitation to feel more, move differently, and connect with yourself and others in new ways. This is my gift to you, so you can embody this new world that is living inside of you right now that wants to be free, alive, and full of radiance!

I pray my story can somehow free you from yours. Let's begin.

Radiantly yours,

Phoebe

Introduction

I sat in meditation in front of my computer camera for a somatic therapy session on Zoom, the only safe way to communicate at the beginning of the pandemic. The healer asked me about a traumatic event that may have affected my spinal column from occiput to sacrum around the age of three.

Without thought, I saw the first image I remember in this body. It was me as a very young child, possibly three years old, being cornered in the kitchen by our bulldog. His eyes met mine as we were on the same level, and he had a ferocious bark. He was mad, but I also felt some kind of pain or anxious energy behind those big brown eyes. I remember not understanding why he was so mad or why I was here in front of him, and I then heard a voice from somewhere beyond that room saying, "This is your first memory." I tried to hold on to the experience and the memory, but it faded. I would occasionally recollect it again as I glimpsed back to my childhood.

I shared this memory with my healer, even though I didn't think it had anything to do with what she requested, but I have learned through numerous healing therapies over the years that everything belongs.

We then traveled to the root of my physical ailments, my reproductive system, and she said there was fear there, a feeling of not being safe. She asked me to relax again and see if anything else came up. I kept thinking in that time and space she was going to ask me more about the dog. Then I kept seeing other dogs: the Doberman we had for only a couple of weeks when I was six years old before my family took him back to the breeder because he was too aggressive towards visitors; Igor, the Beauvoir, that dragged my tiny ten-year-old body across the gravel driveway when I took him for our first walk together; and my last dog Newkie who I was forced to put down amid my divorce because he had a problem biting people.

In the visualization of these memories, she said she saw it wasn't my fear, but my mom's fear that I absorbed and was holding on to. Immediately I saw my mom with me in the corner surrendering to the bulldog, then at the door protecting a visitor from the Doberman, and again the night my pup snapped at her face. She looked at me stunned, not fully knowing he took a chunk of her lip.

I also saw within these flashes from my past my dad cornering my mom and me in the kitchen after throwing two potted plants against the backdoor, another moment when he threw me into the pile of sticks when I wasn't doing my chores, and another time he threw me against the wall when I took the phone from his hand because I thought he was receiving a call from his drug dealer.

What did all of this have to do with what was growing inside of my forty-three-year-old body? What were my body and this string of memories trying to tell me? Moments, which, out of context to this experience, would seem unconnected over time and space, all present inside of me energetically in this instant.

What if we all began to connect our own inner dots and see that something else is going on here beyond what we know to be our reality? What if we became aware that there is something humming underneath, above, within, and all around, that we don't normally choose to see but if we just looked beyond this time and space as we know it, perhaps some mysteries of our own lives will begin to unravel? What if we began to experience a great unfolding of a new reality revealing how everything is connected, everything is happening here and now?

Have you ever felt your gut tell you to do something out of nowhere in an instant that ended up changing the trajectory of your life? Or have you ever made a choice from your heart even though your mind was telling you differently as you contemplated it for days? What if you could listen to your body *and* your intuition with more reverence to make more grounded choices, more creative choices, more innovative choices, more heart-centered choices, more honest choices, more conscious choices, and more connected choices? Did you somewhere along the way stop listening? Do you really know what it means to truly listen to your body? Or are there messages from your body that are getting lost in translation?

We all speak the language of the body before we even learn to speak. Look at babies for example: When they want food, they cry; when they want to be picked up, they reach with their hands; when they want to feel safe, they reach for whoever makes them feel best; when words or music make them happy, their bodies respond with joy, excitement, and movement. But somewhere along the way, we began to learn other languages and our intuitive language got quieter. Adults condition children to sit still and be quiet, though their bodies feel the excitement or the intensity of a situation. Over time, as children, we learn what is expected of us. We want the approval of our adults and deny what we *feel* is the right response. As a result of clamping down on our intuitive responses and shutting off our natural reactions of the nervous system, we forget how to hear them. We lose the ability to feel and listen to the body's signals.

Our Body Knows

I watched David Byrne's *American Utopia* on Hulu the other day. In his opening monologue, he remarks about how babies' brains have hundreds of millions more neural connections than adults, and how as we grow up, we lose those connections. As you can imagine, he goes on to make a joke that we get dumber as we get older. He then shares that we get rid of some of the connections that are not useful, which allows us to get to the core of who we are as a person, who we are in the external world, how we perceive our world, and how to make some kind of sense of it. This got me to contemplate how we have always had these codes of who we are deep within us but are set up to go on an inner journey of self-discovery to reveal the true nature of our being.

A few days later, I discussed with a friend how our body is quite magnificent. She spoke about her experience of having a baby and she said, "It's amazing that my body knows how to make the baby and deliver the baby, but when it gets out into this world, I have no idea what to do with it. That's because my mind gets in the way!" Along with all the "how to" baby books, social media noise from "perfect" moms, and ridiculous expectations set by society that adds to the loud mind chatter, how can she possibly hear her body wisdom speak to her?

Whenever or wherever we lose these intuitive connections, we *can* reclaim them and remember who we are, what makes us happy, and what our souls came here to do.

I align with the Eastern world belief that our souls choose our bodies, our location, our timing, our skin color, our parents, and all the other external factors our souls come into as babies, to then play out the lessons we chose to learn for this life so we can live out our purpose. Here, I share how I found my way through reconciling with this idea.

This is an invitation for you to remember, reconnect with, and reclaim the voice of your body, your intuition, your inner knowing, your soul's calling. You have everything you need right here. Your body is one of your life partners, your breath is another. It is time to look inward and feel safe to listen to it again and watch how the world outside of it unfolds into something beyond magic.

How to Read This Book

Think of this book as an invitation into the dance of discovering yourself again. The first act, *Pas de Deux with Dad*, is my story of the relationship with my dad. I share my own vulnerable story of first mistrusting and denying, then eventually reclaiming my own intuition with the hope of inspiring you to do the same. As you read about my journey, allow yourself to experience what it could have felt like in my body. There might be moments that really speak to you that resonate with your own story, and others that you do not know why you can feel what you feel, but trust it, follow it with curiosity. The second act, *Dark Dances of the Soul,* is a continuation of the specific emotions that arose from these events. These emotions are the ones that we often think of as our shadow emotions or negative feelings. In the third act, *Grand Jeté into the Sun*, we dance in the lighter emotions and examine how they each manifested in my body and my life. There are sections in the last two acts, where we sit together, and I guide you to do some inquiry on how these emotions may show up in your own body and story. I then invite you into expansive awareness and self-inquiry practices that have helped me through my own transformation—I hope they serve you on yours.

ACT ONE

PAS DE DEUX WITH DAD

I used to dance around the living room…
and I'd say, "Daddy, I would *love* to dance."

— *A Chorus Line*

In My Beginning

I was a baby that was just like you, sensitive to my survival needs of eating, sleeping, and wanting to feel safe. In a lot of ways, I chose two extremely loving parents. However, my mom has said that I may have been a bit more sensitive than the average baby because I would cry until I was literally blue in the face. She and my dad thought that I was actually going to cry myself to death a couple of times. Why did this tiny baby that felt so loved cry herself blue? I believe we all are empaths, but some of us just forget it or avoid it as we get older because it is just too hard to handle. Although I was loved by my parents, I lived in a rather chaotic home life and could not help but pick up on the energies that were around me.

My dad was a hippie drug dealer who originally ran his weed business out of his waterbed store protected by two lions that lived on the roof. Yes, that sentence is correct, and no, my dad was not Joe Exotic. It was just the seventies. My dad was always a bit of a wild man and got a bit wilder after his two tours as a helicopter pilot in Vietnam. He seemed to make choices that always had him living on the edge, and when I came along, that put me in a similar place and created a pattern deeply embedded in me well into my adulthood.

He met my mom one day while he was walking one of his lions, Simba, in York, PA. She was at a bus stop waiting to go to class at the nearby college when she saw this handsome man with a lion and decided to flirt with him. The rest of it becomes *my story*.

During our early years together, there was much instability. Dad had steady work for a bit but quickly ended up being out of work after he hurt his back badly from falling off a ladder. He needed money to support us. So, he went back to dealing dope again. First, it was weed but then he went big time with dealing cocaine to the Pagans, a motorcycle gang. Mom would ask these big burly men to, "Please leave your weapons at the door and please be quiet, my baby is asleep in the next room." They would leave their guns at the door as per Mom's request, but they didn't always abide by the latter; thankfully I was generally a good sleeper. I still managed to sleep amidst the rowdy men while they sampled their purchases with Dad which made their conversations even more animated. Mom watched these guys go in and out of our home all hours of the day and night. Being in her young twenties, it was wild and cool until Dad's colleagues started showing up dead in car trunks.

Mom began to feel uneasy and there were times the chaos was taking over their lives altogether. The FBI started following Dad when he got stopped in Florida with a suitcase full of about $20,000 in cash. They busted him shortly after and he cut a deal with them. He told them what they needed to know, and they wiped his slate clean. Dad was a super charming guy when he needed to be; he was also smart, and a veteran, so he somehow cut into the deal with them to move out of the area and go to the trade school of his choice to start a different life. He chose computer school and was good at it. He became a computer programmer and we moved to the suburbs of DC a short time after he got a job offer. My mom learned some computer skills too and she changed her career path from being a Wendy's drive-thru cashier to working for the government at the Office of Technology Assessment. I got to keep her Wendy's uniform for my dress-ups though, which made me very happy. It was a new beginning for our little family to live the typical suburban life. In my little world, this seemed absolutely perfect.

Dad was always a wild man though. He wasn't afraid to put himself and others in dangerous situations. He seemed to get high on it at times. One night when I was still a baby, my parents left me with my gramma during one of their crazy nights out. My gramma still tells me how she thought it was going to just be the two of us from that night on. She wasn't sure if they would ever come back. She was close to right.

That night Mom and Dad were out with some friends, an interracial couple, a white man and a Black woman. Some rednecks began to harass Dad's friends outside of a gas station while getting more beer and cigarettes. Dad decided to stand up for his friends and yelled back, "Go fuck yourself!" This was rural Pennsylvania in the late seventies, I'm still not sure when is the best time to be bold to a group of drunken racists, but that was definitely not the time nor place. Just like out of a scene of a movie, the group of men went to their pickups to draw their rifles. Mom, Dad, their friends, and our bloodhound, Doodah, packed into their car and peeled out of the gas station. It turned into a car chase with gunshots aimed at my parents' car. They hit a ditch and were thrown off the road into the dark country woods. Everyone panicked yet laid low in the car quietly, not moving, praying the crazy clan would pass and not find them. Doodah ran off into the pitch-black night. The car blazed past and didn't show any sign of slowing down. They were safe. They called for Doodah for hours and eventually, he found his way back. When they returned to Gramma's, I lay in the bassinet angelically smiling at my parents, welcoming them home.

I had no idea what type of adventure they had been on, nor should I have. All I needed to know then was that I was simply loved. I felt that. When Dad battled his demons with drinking and drugs, they reared their ugly heads in our home with anger, rage, depression, mania, and violence. I felt that too.

There was a lot of energy that I was picking up on that, as a baby, I didn't quite know how to hold or make sense of in my little body. When I went through Dad's psych reports after his death, I came across an examination that documented an incident he recalled in a session about a time when he couldn't take the demons anymore. He recounted that he pulled out his gun from a drawer, put it to his head, then heard his baby daughter cry out in the next room. He paused for a moment, put the gun away, and went to go check on her. Was that me needing a diaper changed or me crying out for my own dad's life? Although I may never truly know, I like to believe that something within me told me to cry out because I was so very connected to my dad. It was divine timing in the form of a poopy diaper.

My First Teacher and Practices

Dad was probably the biggest instigator of creating the chaotic energy within me and around me but also one of my first teachers in connecting me to the energy of my body and the space. He taught me how to control my energy through breath. As a young child, I got overwhelmed and cried myself to hyperventilation. When Dad was good, he was there to calm me; he would hold me, tell me to breathe, show me how to sit and put my head between my legs, and sometimes offer me to breathe into a paper bag. He would guide me to slow down my breaths and acknowledge how the energy started to slow down and then calm me down. This was a powerful practice for me to utilize alone when Dad wasn't so good, and he was having his own episodes that he seemingly could not control.

I found my way to other practices that kept my mind and body calm when it was hard to contain all the energy of my chaotic life. There were nights I lay in bed, tossing and turning, and somehow intuitively, I flipped a switch on in my "brain vacuum" and watched the thoughts of my day get sucked out from the back of my head into the pillow. I watched each event and each thought disappear, leaving me to sleep peacefully and dream up new possibilities for my life.

If there were any thoughts that were resistant to the suck of the vacuum, I would pull out my little diary and pen, write down all the thoughts and feelings that still lingered, then lock them up. I would then stow away the tiny key in the sugar bowl of the antique tea set I used to host tea parties for my stuffed animals and very special human guests. My thoughts scared me sometimes when I began to realize how powerful they could be, so I felt they needed to be erased or locked up when I sometimes would see a thought unfold in front of my very own eyes. This can be very cool as a kid, yet very disturbing, especially when having thoughts about others that are not so good. As we dive more deeply into my past you will see what I mean.

My greatest practice, by far, was the gift of dance. Mom still says that I danced before I walked because I spent hours in the jolly jumper hopping up and down to the beats of whatever was playing on our record player. It could be Aretha Franklin, Elton John, Stevie Wonder, BB King, The Cars, Blondie, my Uncle Tom's made-up songs about my moony eyes, or Gramma and Aunt June playing "Alley Cat " on their pianos. Whatever it was, I found my way to dance to it. This continued once I got on my own two feet into jazz, tap, and ballet classes, and most nights in front of my parents for a post-dinner dance performance. It brought me so much joy and I believed my dancing brought other people joy too. Even after a long day of work, I'm sure my exclusive performance of the entire *Miss Piggy's Aerobique Exercise Workout Album* made my parents' lives more enlightened and enriched, especially with the showstopper "Snackcercise." I danced at all hours in my room and my basement when I was in rehearsal mode. As I got older and things got more complicated, I danced my way to a place to make sense of my world. It was the one place I felt safe when the outside world was more unpredictable and chaotic. It was a place that opened other worlds for me to connect with and to help me believe there was a way to feel that anything was possible again.

All these practices were gifts, but I didn't realize how much they were until much later in life. When I filled out an application for a yoga teacher training program that asked,

"How long have you been practicing yoga?" I realized, after looking back at my recent history of taking yoga classes, I began to trace back the actual practice all the way back here: breathwork with Dad to calm my anxiety, meditation and contemplation to clear my thoughts, and movement to get my "ya-yas" out, as my yoga teacher, Jeanmarie, would always say in class.

As I reflect on my childhood as an adult, I often wonder who or where I would be without these practices. Would I have followed in the footsteps of Dad being homeless and/or thrown in jail? Would I have shut myself off from feeling my feelings with drugs because of the traumatic events of my childhood? Would I have shut myself out from the possibility of healthy relationships and dream job opportunities because the outside world had abandoned me way too many times? Maybe I will never know, maybe there is another version of me playing those lives out in alternate universes. What I do know is that I am so very grateful I had these practices that saved my life, my inner voice that kept me safe, and those neural pathways that didn't lose their connections.

Reading the Signs

There were so many moments I felt loved unconditionally by my parents. When they were still together and when those times were good, I could always run into a room and get a hug. Often, I would walk in and see my parents snuggling together and I would ask, "Can I join in?" They would open their arms and I would pile on top of the two of them to receive hugs and kisses from them both as if they were just sitting there waiting for me to enter. The nights I woke up from a nightmare, I would cry out from my bed, run to their room quickly to avoid the monsters, and crawl into bed between their warm bodies as a shield from what haunted me in my own bed moments before. I would feel safe again.

In those calm times, I knew that the monsters in my dreams could not get me if Mom and Dad were close. But as I got a bit older, I started to see those nightmares as a reality that I could not wake from, and oftentimes it was my very own Dad who was the monster because his demons were catching up with him. In those moments when I feared him, he could not hold me close, guide me to breathe, and tell me everything would be okay. I had to learn how to watch the signs and plan the swiftest way to safety on my own. I had to learn how to find my own way out of that darkness and find a new path to the light. I soon learned my parents would not always be there to guide me in the spaces of chaos. It was all up to me to feel the energy and figure out the best way to stay safe.

My Stories

The Last Valentine's Day

This Valentine's evening was a typical February evening, cold and dreary, but Daddy's warm heart came into my room and lit me up, as he always did. He brought all of us gifts for this very special day; for Mom and my aunt who was living with us, he gave potted plants, and for me, the biggest Valentine's card ever and an I Love You balloon.

Daddy's note said how much he loved me and how proud he was of me. He had the most beautiful and unique penmanship; he had a very curvy and expressive way of writing, always in all capitals, and with his special red felt pen. He wrote everything with that pen, from his little Post-it notes to every official document and bill, to my Valentine's Day envelope with his doodled hearts all over it. Hearts were his thing. He drew hearts for me everywhere. I kept the balloon roaming free until it lost its last breath of air, then I pinned it next to my card on my wall for years as a reminder of Dad's love and one of the last days of my childhood innocence.

After Dad gave me a big hug to accompany my Valentine's Day gifts, he announced he was taking Mom and me out for dinner to one of my favorite places, Victoria Station, a restaurant made from old train cars. It was super fancy, and we always got to go there for special occasions like Valentine's Day or when I got good grades on my report card. I got dressed up in my favorite red and white dress and my white stockings with red hearts on them to match the occasion. We ate, they drank, I got dessert and Dad ordered his favorite drink, Tia Maria with coffee. I felt so warm and beamed even in the dead of the cold winter because I was so loved by my parents.

As we drove home though, the energy shifted, Dad seemed agitated. He began to drive much faster with abandon and the music became unbearably loud. I asked to have it turned down because it hurt my ears, but neither of my parents could hear me up front since they were now starting to talk louder at each other. I sat helplessly in the back seat covering my ears and started to shiver. Suddenly, I just wanted to be home in my own bed, under the covers to find warmth, and to hide from the tense energy I was feeling coming from the front of the car.

When we got home, things got really blurry, as if I put myself to sleep to escape a nightmare. I went somewhere else. I can't explain what happened next but when I came to, I was crouched in the kitchen corner with Mom. She was shaking, and her tears were soaking my hair as she had her arms around me. I looked across the room where I would normally sweep after dinner every night, and there was Dad standing over a pile of dirt, broken pottery, and the remains of the plants he gave Mom and my aunt as gifts just hours before. There was dirt on the door and walls next to where he stood. All had been broken. Those plants, my family, and me. I felt like my world was dismembered—my dad on one side of the room, so disconnected, my mom's arms around me but not holding me, and me, who felt just like those plants that were under my dad's feet now—crushed.

Dad looked back at us with red hot eyes, maybe he was still mad, or maybe he just woke up from my nightmare too. Then he just walked away; he went upstairs to his study like nothing happened. Mom peeled away from me to clean up the mess and she sent me to bed. We never spoke of that night again.

The Valentine's Day card hung on my wall for years as a bittersweet reminder of that night. From then on, I found myself consciously tuning into the signs of any rumblings of danger below the surface. What I thought to be solid ground was no longer stable. For survival, I kept myself aware and quickly learned when to flee to a safe place.

And Then There Were Two

A couple of months later, on a Saturday afternoon, Mom and I went to run her errands, one of them being a stop at the bank. As she took a big wad of cash and my lollipop out from the tube sent over from the teller at the drive-thru, she said something that caught my attention. She said something to the effect that there were going to be big changes in our family soon. My heart sank a bit because her tone did not sound like a good change, my mind started to race through possibilities to prepare myself. *Are we moving again? Will I have to change schools and make new friends again?* It did not seem like it was the time to ask questions, so I just got quiet and observed.

The next day, she sat me down in the front yard and told me she was leaving Dad. It didn't fully sink in yet that because she was leaving my dad, I was no longer going to be with my mommy and daddy together. I asked her if she could stay with me in my home and if I could stay in the same school. She did not give me a straight answer. She went inside to speak with Dad.

I stayed outside as they were inside discussing our future—my future—something I never had to think about up until that moment. I did not know what that future would look like, but it was sinking in that it would no longer include the three of us, the only thing I had ever known up until that point. My world was collapsing. Until that moment, I always felt so incredibly loved and I was worried I would no longer feel that way ever again.

As the sun began to set and the fireflies started to light up my front yard, which was happening more frequently as a sign of summer coming, I just sat still. I did not leap up and try to chase them like I usually did with little sounds of glee bursting out of me. At this point in the evening, Mom usually asked me to come inside and get ready for bed and I would delay it so I could be free with the little light show that danced in front of me.

That evening, I sat there. All those memories of the three of us would soon become fragmented then replaced with lonely weekday dinners with Dad and fun-filled weekends to cover up the sadness with Mom and her soon-to-be new boyfriend. The happy memories of the three of us would perhaps forever be distorted. In my mind, I quickly tried to capture those blissful memories of us together like my fireflies in a jar to keep them from flying away from me. But like anything that is captured, they would soon die anyway. One by one those moments would shine their last burst of light and drop to the bottom of the jar. There was no use. Our family, my family, was broken forever. My heart would be shattered for a very long time and the scars, deep.

Mom returned to tell me the news. She was moving out and I would stay in the house with Dad to continue the life I knew. I would still go to my school and play with my friends. I was relieved in knowing my daily life would stay the same, but it did not quite hit me yet that the void I would soon know well would feel like carrying a heavy load without an essential leg.

Mom tucked me into bed, and she left our home after I fell asleep. The next day, I somehow managed to wake up without the sound of Mom's voice saying, "Phoebe, time to get up!" Perhaps Dad woke me, I do not quite remember. However I woke up, it was so very foreign but I recognized I had to claim a new normal. On my way out the door, Dad handed me a note to give to my second-grade teacher, Mrs. Patrick. It was written on a yellow legal pad with his red felt pen but this time his penmanship was a little shaky. As he handed it to me, he looked me in the eyes and said, "If you need anything, don't be afraid to tell them to call me, you hear me? Anything. I will come get you. I love you, hun." I nodded my head as I shook off my pain. I told myself I had to be a big girl now and get through the day. We hugged tightly, as we always did, and we both did our best to hold back the tears that so badly wanted to burst from our eyes.

When I walked into my classroom, all my friends came rushing up to me so joyfully telling me about their weekend adventures with their families. Like a warrior, I focused on my task. I walked through the bubble of happiness and glee and single-handedly burst it as I handed my teacher the note with my little shaky hand. For some reason, this was the biggest moment of not turning back. Before, there was a chance Mom would come back, but now, it was written words on a paper that my teacher would read and somehow declare to the world as a fact. As if the rest of the class was also reading this yellow legal paper with the red felt pen writing on it, the whole room shifted and looked at me in deafening silence as Mrs. Patrick read the note that said my family was now broken and my dad would be the point of contact if his little girl needed anything that day or any other day from then on. He signed his name and his work phone number. My teacher looked at me with pity and asked if I was okay. I nodded but then I began to cry. It was the first time I cried since I heard the news. Between sobs buried in my teacher's lap, I could hear the whispers of my classmates asking, "What is wrong with Phoebe?" and the replies, "I think her mommy left her daddy."

The next couple of weeks were a blur, with interspersed phone calls from Mom to see how I was holding up. I somehow managed school and as soon as the second grade was over, Dad shipped me to my Uncle Barry's in Michigan. I stayed with him, his wife, and their dog, Shithead. It was not a fun place, but I guess it was not as gloomy as home. I did not know much about my uncle up until then except he smoked cigarettes, he was a heart doctor, and he drove a fancy car called a Corvette. I also felt that there was some kind of competition between my uncle and my dad that I did not quite understand, and I was a little uneasy around him, especially when he laughed which was very loud, explosive, and kind of creepy. During my time in Michigan, I learned that my uncle took about six different vitamins with every meal, he liked split pea soup, and he expected me to like split pea soup too.

When I returned home, I began to see Mom again. She and Dad worked out visitation rights in court that consisted of Mom coming to see me one night a week at my home for an hour or two while Dad was in the house; he always disappeared upstairs though, and Mom was not allowed to take me out of the house the first few visits together. The first time she came to visit, I didn't want to see her. I didn't want to see her at all that whole summer. We sat at the dining room table. I sat in her old chair. It was my chair now. I had taken it over after she left. She struggled to have a conversation with me. She asked me questions, and I gave her the shortest answers possible and did not look at her. I wanted to tell her how unhappy Dad was and how our home was now covered with a veil of sorrow. I wanted to tell her that he cried into my lap after dinner every night and claimed I was his only family now. I was so mad at her, but I let it simmer inside of me to bathe in it all alone. I could not tell her because I didn't feel like I could trust her anymore. All I wanted was for someone to take away my pain and I knew it could not be my mom and dad anymore since they were both already carrying a huge load of pain of their own.

Flashback

Dad and I were doing our best to keep things normal. We had a Saturday ritual of cleaning the house together. I was always in charge of dusting and vacuuming the stairs. Dad would put on his favorite radio program, *The Bama Hour,* which featured an old Black man with a slow southern drawl and a crackly voice that shared depressing stories about heartbreak. Then after a long monologue, he would play these old songs by artists who sang their tales of loss and sadness where you could hear the needle move over the grooves of the album as if they were playing over the singers' heartbreaks and emotional scars. This music was called the blues, and man, they got deep into the waters of sorrow and bathed there for probably years until they were well beyond pruned up. These stories usually began with, "My baby left me..." Yeah, I could relate to their pain.

Despite the depressing music in the background, it was a beautiful day, and I enjoyed this Saturday ritual with Dad. We had the doors and windows wide open to let in all the light and clear out the stagnant air. It was my day to see Mom, but I didn't want to. I didn't want to leave Dad, he actually seemed happy for the first time, and I didn't want to go with her. I was still mad at her for leaving us.

The stereo was cranked up and the vacuum roared. I heard a faint ringing of the phone in the background, over and over again. I knew it was Mom. Dad didn't seem to hear it, so I pretended to not hear it either. Shortly after the phone stopped ringing, I saw Mom'scar pull up to my home and she began to walk up the walkway to our door. In a split second, everything changed.

Suddenly, Dad went down a rabbit hole and took all of us with him. As Mom approached the wide-open front door, Dad slammed it on her arms several times to get it to shut and keep her out. She cried out, "Jay, it's me, Brenda! I'm here to see Phoebe! Jay! It's my day to see Phoebe!"

He screamed a bunch of things at her I didn't quite understand. After moments of struggling and pushing her, he managed to get her limbs out of the door, then he slammed it closed and locked it, both the deadbolt and the chain, then, with his back to the door, he slid down to sit and pressed his whole-body weight against it to be sure she could not get in. Once he felt the door was securely locked, he yelled at me to lay low while he ran into his bedroom. I was huddled in the kitchen, in the same place Mom and I had crouched together with the dismembered plants months before, while I observed the scene in front of me. I was in shock and felt so disconnected from my body and from the two people I loved most. I wasn't sure if I was even in my own body or watching two characters I barely knew in a movie. The next few moments were filled with even more chaos. Mom rang the doorbell and banged on the door over and over again and cried to see me while Dad paced back and forth from the living room to his bedroom. He then told me to get ready, scooped me up, ran with me over his shoulder out the back door, around the house, and threw both of us into his car. He screeched down the driveway and Mom ran to her car to follow us. I was now in the middle of a car chase with my two parents, who were fighting over me. At some point in the next town over, we lost her at the traffic light of a major intersection. I watched her car get smaller and smaller. For the first time, I missed my mommy and wished I was with her in her car so she could drive me far away from the madness. I had no idea where we were headed next.

We arrived at a familiar apartment complex. It was Dad's friend Jim's place. Dad took deep breaths when he parked the car. When we walked into Jim's, Dad handed him a gun and said, "Man, keep this away from me. I got really close to using it today."

The rest of the afternoon was spent at Jim's in a cloud of pot smoke while they passed a bong and took hits back and forth while I watched TV and tried to find my way back to my body and recover from the day's events.

Tiny Dancer

Ever since I could remember, I danced. I danced in classes, with friends, with family members, outside under the big blue sky, in my little bedroom, in dress-up costumes, and in just underwear.

Dance has always been the one place where I could truly honestly be just me. As a child, it was my outlet to be free. I could move however I wanted, to whatever music I wanted, tell whatever stories I wanted, feel anything and everything I wanted, and create whatever world I wanted. You see, when I danced, magic happened. My dreams became realities for me there. Later, as I went out into the world and found out life wasn't as exciting as it was in the dances I created, I was a bit disillusioned by this realm we call *reality*.

When I danced in my room alone, I was connected to something much bigger than myself. I felt so connected to that radiant being that we all are. I felt the radiance deep in my soul but as a child, it was hard to conceptualize. Through movement, I created worlds where I was dancing for people who watched my every move outside my window. They always seemed in awe of my beauty and grace, especially when I got back up again from a fall. I was so pleased to dance for them and share my gift. I was always a little sad when real people came to see me in my shows when I started to perform as a professional. I didn't feel like they saw me like the unworldly spirits that watched me in my room as a child. I felt like they weren't awake; they didn't get it. It was heartbreaking to witness them. If only they could see what I was expressing. Not from an egotistical place but from a place where they were missing something inside of themselves, like I was trying to show them a secret about their own radiance that they had forgotten.

Dancing for Dad

Dad always got home from work by the end of *Oprah*. I would watch Oprah share people's inspirational stories of strength and resilience. Perhaps it helped me juggle the chaos at home. Dad would immediately change from his work clothes to his comfy clothes, which consisted of the worn-in pale blue jeans that he probably had as long as I was alive and a blue and yellow long-sleeved polo shirt.

Dad would make dinner for the two of us and I did my best to finish what was on my plate to please him. Every night, I would sit on the edge of my seat (literally) bounce and wiggle around, ready to take off to the next thing that was on my metaphorical plate while I ate. I was such a wiggler that when Dad went to get the antique dining chairs rewoven, he had to get the whole frame redone because the left side was completely worn out where my tiny butt had created a whole new indentation from all the movement.

Most nights after dinner, I was allowed to put on a show. Honestly, this is what got me through dinner and that entire period of my life. Our dining room opened to the living room with a subtle archway, just enough to give the illusion of a proscenium stage. I would already have my costumes preset backstage, or rather, the part of the living room that was not visible from the dining room. I would cue Dad to turn the music on, his only production job, and then he was to be the audience.

Post-dinner shows were my time to shine! Dancing was the one thing that no one could ever take away from me back then. It was my therapy, my love, my freedom, my joy. It was just simply mine.

The show would begin. I would take the stage and Dad watched—except he was the rudest audience member ever. He talked to me through the performances all the time, a really big no-no in audience etiquette. I tried to teach him that it was rude to speak to the performers, but he would not listen, I would say, "DAD! Just watch me dance! You can't talk during a show!" And he would keep on going, blah, blah, blah. He sat there on his chair, rolling his cigarettes, and say, "I love you so much, hun. I believe in you. You are so talented. You can do anything you want to do. Really! Believe it! Don't let anyone tell you differently, and if they do, tell them to eat shit, and die! And if anyone ever fucks with you, you tell me, and I will kill those assholes." Yeah, words of affirmation and wisdom from my dad, Jay R. Miller III.

I don't know if I ever really heard him until many years later. I don't know when or why I started to believe differently.

After the performance, Dad's talks would get more and more serious and more ominous. Sometimes, many times, he started crying and I had to comfort him. I would then sit in his chair, the head of the table, with his head in my lap as he wept and said, "You are my only family, hun."

A New Girl in Our Home

By the end of the third grade, Dad started dating after he learned Mom had also moved on. He had a new girlfriend, Katie. She was 25, Dad was 40. I didn't really get it. I never quite trusted her; she was very immature and dramatic. There were numerous times she would have hysterical fits and break up with Dad, then days later show up on our doorstep as if nothing happened. She moved in with us early on and made big changes in our world. Katie made Dad tear up our dark green carpets and refinish the hardwood floors that were underneath. She redecorated our home, so things were generally a lot lighter, which was nice. Katie also updated Dad's wardrobe with new light gray Reeboks and brighter colored shirts of my favorites, pink and purple. He didn't seem to mind the changes. In fact, I think he really liked them.

There was a night when I was feeling a bit nervous about Dad's drinking. Katie and Dad drank a lot together, which was not good for Dad. Mom had told me that was why she left him. She said that alcohol was his trigger for getting mad at her. I saw how scary he could be that day with the gun, and I found my ways of coping, but it was starting to weigh on me. Katie sensed something was wrong and took me for a walk to the circle where we sat on benches and started talking about meaningless things. She then started to get more serious and ask questions about my happiness, my mom, and my dad.

Katie somehow got it out of me that I was scared of Dad when he drank and that Mom left Dad because of his drinking problem. The moment the words left my lips I regretted them. I begged and pleaded with her not to tell Dad. She ran her fingers through my hair, held me, kissed me on the head, and said, "Of course. Your secret's safe with me, Phoebe." The way she touched me always made me feel uncomfortable. My body shivered like I was cold, and my stomach always held a fist inside when she came close to me. I always felt like she had a hidden agenda. I never felt what she said or the gestures that she made were ever genuine.

It wasn't even five minutes after we got home that she went into the room where Dad was drinking and watching TV and told him everything I had just shared with her in confidence. He started yelling my name and busted through the door into my bedroom, with his red-hot eyes of rage, he started screaming at me, "You think I have a fucking drinking problem?!? I will show you a fucking drinking problem!" He threatened me and then left the room to get the phone. He paced back and forth down the hallway outside of my bedroom while he screamed into the phone at Mom. I don't know all of what he said because I had a pillow over my head as I tried to get rid of the nightmare I had somehow just created with my words. I knew better by then about who to trust and how not to set him off. Why was this happening?

When Monday morning came, Dad started the process for divorce from Mom after a year of separation. It became clear why it was happening. Katie got what she wanted, a divorced version of Dad who would months later propose to her.

A Christmas Flashback

It was nearing Christmas and I was in the fourth grade. Dad and Katie were still together.

The Christmas tree was all lit up and the presents for me were stacked underneath. I had probably already unwrapped my presents to get a sneak peek of my gifts and re-taped them so no one would know I peeked like I always did. I was always too excited for surprises.

Dad and Katie were newly engaged and had a few friends over to celebrate the season. People mingled between the living room, dining room, and kitchen. Dad was in the kitchen. Katie and I were in the living room sitting in the glow of the tree. By this time, Katie was slurring her words; she turned the music up and started singing the drunker she got. The energy shifted quickly, and I felt more uncomfortable being around her. During these times when they drank, I usually hid in my room but that night it was hard to hide with the people there. Katie leaned into me like she was telling me a secret but spoke loudly in my ear. She put her arms around me, I tried wiggling away from her and said, "Let me go!" All of a sudden, time cracked open, and everything went into slow motion. Dad suddenly appeared from the other room, wedged himself between the two of us, pushed her away from me, and hit her. Katie ran out the front door; for some reason I followed. Dad ran after us and pushed me out of the way into the bushes right outside our front door. He lunged at her, jumped on her, and continued to pummel her. Their friends stood there in shock. She was crying and trying to crawl away from Dad. It all happened so fast, yet everything was still in slow motion as I watched each blow to Katie's face. Someone grabbed me and put me in my bedroom. I don't know what happened after that.

When I woke up the next day, it was just Dad and me in the house. There was never a mention of what happened the night before or where Katie went or if she was coming back. The next weekend was my weekend with Mom. As we drove our regular route through DC to her apartment in Mt. Pleasant, she very cautiously asked me if anything strange had happened at home the weekend before. She wanted to know if everything was okay and if I needed to tell her anything. I didn't know what to say so I said everything was fine. She told me she'd had lunch with Katie and that her face was pretty beat up. Katie came to tell Mom that Dad did it and that Mom should take me away from him. I told her that she was mistaken. I told her that Katie was a crazy drunk and was being dramatic. I even made a weak attempt to tell a story about my theory of how she got the bruises and scars.

I had no real reason to lie but I watched myself do it. Part of me sat in the backseat yelling, "Phoebe! Why are you lying to your mom! Tell her! She already knows anyway!!!"

I had never told a real lie before, only white lies, which were okay because those didn't hurt people, and Mom even knew when I was attempting to tell those kinds of lies. *Did I fool her this time?*

I had no real rational explanation for lying except that I was Dad's only family and that I had to stay. In my mind, I convinced myself that it was a white lie to keep Dad from getting hurt or from him hurting someone else. I couldn't rat him out, he had protected me from Katie, and I could not have him taken away from me because of that. Something kept telling me I was the motivating force that calmed him and gave him a purpose to take care of something bigger than himself.

A few days later, Katie came back to our doorstep, the cuts and bruises that Dad had given her the week before, still on her face. They stayed engaged for a little while longer and then she left for good within a year or so.

Left Alone

The middle school years got a bit more chaotic at my home. While other kids at that age loathed school, maybe even preferred to stay home under the covers to hide from the awkwardness of their changing bodies and worlds, I thrived as long as I wasn't at home. Between dancing, being captain of poms, getting the lead in the school play, and my discovery of boys I was able to stay sane during those wonder years.

Dad was single again and would occasionally have sleepovers with his girlfriends and they would jump on their bed together late at night (at least that is what I thought they were doing back then, and I didn't understand why they were allowed to while I was not).

We began renting out one of our bedrooms on the second floor to a couple of different single women to cover the mortgage which seemed to be getting more challenging for Dad to handle on his own. Most of the roommates were nice except the last one we had; Janice was not nice. She and Dad got into nasty screaming fights which made things even more intense in my house.

At this point, I had moved into the other upstairs bedroom, and I became more accustomed to hiding from the household drama most nights and talking up my fun version of drama on the phone with my girlfriends. We usually talked about who was going to the Friday night dances, who we wanted to dance with, then debrief after the dances to get the full report on who we danced with, how we danced with them (either hands around the neck like proper sixth graders or full bodies pressed up together like eighth graders), who kissed who, and any other important gossip coverage we needed to address to prepare ourselves for the next week of school.

One Friday night I came home from the dance super happy because I got to dance with an eighth grader, Ryan Caden (I was only in sixth, so it was pretty cool). I was ready to run upstairs and write all about the night in my journal: what he smelled like (Old Spice!), how close he held me (our bodies pressed up like eighth graders!), and what song we danced to (Guns n 'Roses, "Every Rose Has its Thorn").

My passionate diary session was put on pause when Dad and I saw a cop car parked at our home. Dad slowed down and continued to drive past our house and down our street but then decided to turn back around at the traffic circle. When we walked into my house, there was a police officer in my living room talking with a hysterical Janice. She was screaming at the police officer to arrest Dad because he was crazy, and that he was doing and dealing drugs out of our house. I didn't quite understand what was happening and started crying. I pleaded to the officer that *she* was crazy and that Dad didn't do drugs. I told the officer my dad was very loving and supportive, that he even helped me with my student anti-drug campaign, DARE, which I was a part of at school. Dad didn't say much, in fact he was eerily quiet, which was a bit odd since he was usually outspoken especially if someone was talking shit. The officer finally told Janice she needed to find another home instead of picking fights with her landlord and calling the police. I felt like white trash, like I was living in a scene from the show *COPS* which had just started airing that year. It would have been truly mortifying if a camera crew was with these cops; my life as I knew it would have been over.

The cop left, Janice went to her room in a huff, and Dad ran into his study, and locked himself in the room that had been my old bedroom just months before. Suddenly, I was left in the dark living room alone trying to make sense of what just happened. There was no way I sensed this scene unfolding like the others I witnessed. I was pretty confused by the whole thing, especially since the hint of Old Spice was still on my shirt from the last dance I shared with Ryan. I was still too high from my experience at the dance. How could I be straddling such different worlds?

I went to Dad's door and asked to come in. No answer. It was locked. I began to cry and pleaded for him to let me in. Nothing. I didn't understand what was happening. I got louder and louder with every sob, "Dad, please. Let me in. I don't understand what is going on. Dad?? Dad?? Dad, please, I am scared! Please, Dad!! I just need a hug. Please?" Still nothing. Dead silence. I sat curled up in a little ball leaning on his door. I must have cried myself to sleep there. At some point I woke up and went to my bedroom. His door still locked me out from knowing the truth.

When I got upstairs, I wrote in my journal about my night at the school dance with Ryan, the eighth grader, to try to shift my energy to a different place so I could go back to sleep peacefully. I barely even mentioned the visit from the cop or Dad abandoning me as I sat crying outside his door. I needed to focus on what was real, what was important, what made sense, what I knew to be true in my little world. My reality, my truth, was the smell of Old Spice on Ryan's blue and white striped button-up shirt as we danced close, our bodies intimately touching, making me shiver with butterflies in my stomach; I had never been so close to a boy before; and how the skin on his neck felt when I touched just above the collar of his shirt. I started to obsessively think of Ryan when my thoughts wandered to the confusion of my home life. I found great comfort knowing we would pass each other in the hall every day after fifth and sixth periods and that there might be a chance he would see me and say something or even just make eye contact. It became my mission to make sure he didn't forget about me and have him ask me to dance again.

Heartbroken

During the summers, my gramma would have off from teaching and we would make an annual trip up to Western Pennsylvania where my family was from. We would make obligatory visits to the older family members in Johnstown, PA who shared their latest news about surgeries and family gossip that was deeply embedded with pain and suffering from years, maybe even generations, past. There were no iPhones to distract me and keep me from hearing their stories, so I always sat politely listening, hoping I was learning something from all of this, even if it was just to never get old.

Our final stop was always my Uncle Tom's, Gramma's big brother. We would stay there for a few days, sometimes a week. I always loved going there and being close to him.

His wife, Aunt Pat had an elderly mom who had Alzheimer's. She usually sat in the corner of the living room just watching us. Sometimes she would shuffle around the house. Occasionally she would accuse me of stealing her dog that had died long ago.

One day, it was just the creepy old lady in the corner, Gramma, and me in the house. Gramma was in the kitchen making us lunch and I was in the living room attempting to play the piano, while the older woman was quietly judging me from her spot. The phone rang. The energy shifted with the first ring. Gramma picked it up with a big, bright "Hello!" I could hear the little, mumbling voice in the other line was a female voice that sounded like Mom. Gramma's voice got quiet and didn't say much but a few, "uh, huhs" and bleak questions I couldn't quite make sense of. I played a little less and quieter so I could make out what they were talking about. She hung up the phone. It was silent. I knew something happened. She walked into the living room and sat on the piano bench with me. She held my hand and put it in her lap.

Dad had suffered a heart attack. My own heart exploded, heat rushed through my entire body and then I quickly went numb, it sounded like my head was underwater. She kept talking but I could only hear the echoes of her voice reciting the story she had just heard from Mom. He was home alone at night when he felt the pains in his chest, and he called 911. The ambulance picked him up and took him to the hospital. He was having surgery and would be in the hospital until they knew he would be okay.

I immediately felt guilty that I was not there with him. His only family should have been with him. There was nothing I could do except go to the basement where I slept and had space to be alone to cry. I felt so helpless. I pictured Dad on the couch in my old bedroom, his study, the room he locked himself in that night I cried myself to sleep months before. He usually fell asleep there working or watching TV and then stumbled across the hall into his bed. I saw him wake up holding his chest, struggling to get to the phone and get the words out of his mouth that he needed help. I wondered how the paramedics got into our house, *was he able to walk to the front door and let them in or did they break in?* My mind played out the moments that got him to the hospital over and over and how it would have been different had I been there.

When Uncle Tom came home from work, I heard his jolly steps and his eager Santa-like happy hellos to everyone, then some whispering, then silence. It was all happening just above my head in the kitchen. Shortly after, footsteps came down the stairs to my room. It was Uncle Tom checking in on me. He was wearing a white Hanes undershirt and slacks from work. He sat on my bed and pulled me close, I leaned my head on his big belly that felt like my own pillow as I cried. My little body shook, and his white t-shirt absorbed my anxious sweat and tears. He just let me cry for a little while and held that space for me to feel my sad, mad, confused feelings.

After a long pause, he told me a story. He shared about a son he once had, Michael. I never got to meet him because he died at a very young age. It was devastating for my uncle and the rest of the family to watch his innocent son get so sick. He told me how mad he got that God took away his little boy, but he found a way to overcome it. He believed things always happen for a reason. When he was in a very dark place, he had to find his way out. He was determined to figure out why his little boy got sick and dedicated his life to research to find a cure so other families would not lose their children to that illness. He told me about how he was building a lab in his new home that they would be moving into soon. My Uncle Tom was the smartest man I ever knew; if there was a cure, he would find it.

His story taught me a lot and framed how I would keep going from then on. No matter how bad things would get, I had to know it was always happening for a reason, perhaps to help others in the long run. He was given that life circumstance because he was strong and capable of moving from it to a better place. I would vow to grow from my life circumstances too, and whatever came of them I would always be better because of them.

A couple of days later, Gramma and I made our way back to Rockville to see Dad, we went directly to the hospital. We walked down the sterile hallway and saw a man in a room that looked like him, his weak body dressed in a hospital gown, sitting in a wheelchair next to his bed, hooked up to machines. His voice confirmed it was Dad. He was irritable and yelling at a nurse about how he was crawling out of his own skin and that he was ready to "go the fuck home!" He began to pull the IV out of his arms and tear away all the other devices that he was hooked up to. The machines started beeping loudly. The nurses tried to subdue him, but he was pissed. He calmed down a little bit when he saw me. I was so scared to see him like that. I had never been in a hospital before, let alone visited someone I love. I sat with him for a bit, and we were both uncomfortable. My body was shaking uncontrollably. Even though it was the swampy DC August heat outside, my body could not get warm because of my nerves and the ridiculous hospital air conditioning that was set to "frozen" in case patients died was my guess (perhaps it was safer that way). I could imagine why his skin was crawling after being there for just a few minutes. He told me he wanted a cigarette and that the food was so horrible it upset his stomach.

Nana and Grandpa, his parents, were there too and had been staying in our home. Nana was cleaning the house from top to bottom and rearranging things to her approval. It was her way to keep herself distracted, I guess. During all this, she somehow managed to make me feel guilty for not keeping the house as clean and up to her standards, as a twelve-year-old.

When Dad came home from the hospital, he gave me a VHS tape. It was a recording of his surgery. He got it from the doctor to show me because he thought it was very educational. I never watched it. That just seemed way too odd and gross. That was Dad though. He always wanted me to learn something and open my world to greater possibilities.

The remainder of the summer he rested and got stronger so he could go back to work. In the evenings, we sat out in our front yard, and I watched him roll his cigarettes like he always did, no heart attack was going to take that away from him. He told me how beautiful I was, that I didn't need to cut bangs to cover up my face (even though I begged to have them since all my friends were getting them that summer), or that I didn't need to wear make-up, and that I was so smart that I could be anything I wanted to be, even a doctor if I wanted. I sat and watched the last of the fireflies light up our yard while I listened to him, but I didn't quite hear him until much later in life.

Holding it Together

Shortly after Dad's heart attack, he went back to work, and I began seventh grade. For the next two years, the energy continued to shift in my house. There seemed to be more secrets lurking in the shadows around strange phone calls from a guy who constantly called asking for Dad. During my nightly calls with friends, my call waiting would beep incessantly, from what I imagined was a rather big Black man, named Dwayne. He always wanted me to give Dad a message that he needed to call him back right away. If I didn't pick up, he would call again and again until I gave in. Sometimes I passed it on, but other times I just ignored it simply because I was a tween and was so absorbed in my universe. Something also told me it wasn't safe for Dad to know Dwayne was calling. Dad always had to go run an errand after he called, no matter what time it was. Sometimes he did not come back until I was already in bed.

I came home from school once or twice and my TV was no longer in my room, not because I was grounded from TV for a week like my best friend, Gabby often was. No, I was never in trouble and never had to be punished. My TV was gone because Dad had to "lend it" to one of his "friends" for a little while, but he would get it back.

His "friend" also left messages on our answering machine when we were gone that usually said, "Hey Jay, call me back." There were a few that got angrier tones as time went along. One day Dad's new girlfriend Linda, who was living with us, heard one of the longer and angrier messages and she moved out the next day. I don't know what it said but she left a note warning me to get out too. I never saw her or heard from her again.

During this period, Dad also seemed to be grumpier and moved more quickly from agitated to full-on rage. I avoided making eye contact and talking to him regularly. He still called me from work after I got home from school to make sure I got home safely. He told me what he would make us for dinner and always say, "I love you, hun." Sometimes he made it home for dinner, but when he did, we usually ate in our separate bedrooms. I began to hesitate to say "I love you" back before hanging up the phone. There were even occasions I hung up before he could tell me. I didn't really like who he was anymore or the consistently crappy home life that he was creating for me. I was beginning to resent him.

By the end of eighth grade, he had to put our house on the market. It seemed to be too much for Dad all alone. The whole reason I ended up living with Dad when Mom left was to stay in my home, and the time was coming I would have to move out—another reason I began to resent him.

I was determined to keep the darkness of my home life separate from my bright shiny outer life; I did this by overachieving. By the time I finished middle school I felt pretty accomplished. I was popular with lots of great friends (really! I was lucky I had wonderful friends!); I left middle school as co-captain of the poms squad, was an honor roll student, had a couple of boys who liked me, and to end my days at middle school I played the lead role of Sandy, and choreographed our school version of *Grease*. Dad didn't make it to any of the performances. Secretly, I was glad because I was nervous he might embarrass me since he was having more and more extreme mood swings. Looking back though, I wish he had been there to see me, his little girl, perform on stage.

Unlike most kids entering high school, I felt confident that I was going to rock it there too. Nothing was going to hold me back from succeeding if I could keep my home life separate. However, it lurked in the shadows, and it felt like there were too many close calls.

During that summer between middle and high school, Dad sat me down for a long talk. He told me he had a drug problem and he had struggled with it from the time he was my age, fourteen. He also told me to never start because when you start you stunt your growth and never grow up emotionally from that age. He said that in a way we were the same age, emotionally. I wholeheartedly believed him.

He told me he was going to an outpatient rehab and needed to attend meetings called AA (Alcoholics Anonymous) and that he thought it would be a good idea for me to go along with him and learn more about it. Most of that summer was spent at these meetings with Dad. Sometimes he would go and sit in one room, and I would go and sit in another with other kids who had parents dealing with the same disease. Except it didn't sound like their parents loved them, not as my dad did, and there was much more anger and resentment towards their parents. Perhaps it was my wake-up call to address the resentment that had been building over the last couple of years. It was all very depressing to me. People shared stories but no one had any sound advice or answers to their helpless questions. Instead, it seemed like an empty space for people to dump their sorrows and fester those negative feelings into more heartache. Dad never shared, at least when I was there. I never shared in my group either. It just didn't feel right.

Dad made small triumphs the first few weeks and would come home with a new chip for his number of days of sobriety. Sometimes, he would give me his chip for us both to celebrate it. I was really proud of him. However, he began to stumble with relapses. Each time it got a little worse and more heartbreaking. In a way, it was easier when I didn't really know what was going on.

Towards the end of the summer, I came home from a weekend with Mom and her husband; they both dropped me off. Dad locked himself in the house and would not let me in. He had a relapse and was having some kind of nervous breakdown. He was paranoid. He kept screaming that he had a gun to his head, and it would be better if we just left. Mom did not react to his words; she was convinced he was too scared to face his demons in death. We sat outside my home for what seemed to be hours. Neighbors walked by and quietly judged us. I cried and begged Dad to come out. I told him how proud I was for doing all that he had done so far in his recovery and not to give up. Finally, we somehow got him to open the door and he let me in. We all gathered up his things and took him to the hospital where he entered in-patient rehab, the same hospital he was in just a year earlier for his heart attack. That was the first time Dad met Matt, Mom's husband. We all sat together, the four of us, in the hospital waiting room like it was a normal thing to do. At some point, I excused myself to go make a couple of calls to my friends on the payphone. We had plans to meet that day. About an hour later, I hugged Dad goodbye and he disappeared behind the hospital doors to the drug recovery floor, where he would be for the next two weeks. Mom and Matt drove me to the baseball game where my boyfriend was playing, and I met my girlfriends as originally planned. I laughed with them as if nothing happened earlier that day.

I have no idea how I was able to pull that off; those moments of straddling the two worlds were starting to get to me. How was I going to pull it off when I went to high school? How was Dad going to be after rehab? From that moment, I pushed my feelings aside and just kept moving forward with a smile. I could not let these worlds collide.

Things Fall Apart

When high school began, I was on new turf and was ready to shine. By the time Homecoming came around, the quarterback of the football team asked me to the Homecoming Dance. Dad wasn't there to see me, his little girl, go off to her first high school Homecoming dance. He didn't come home at all that weekend.

I didn't know what to do about Dad. He had been relapsing more and more. I felt it was my responsibility to hold him accountable. I didn't know how to confront him or if it was even safe. I was also concerned that my friends would begin to know something was up. My new older and cooler high school friends drove and would often stop by unannounced to hang out with me. It was harder to protect my outer world reputation. My worlds were beginning to collide. It was hard to explain why my dad wasn't around and worse; when he was around, he was super high, and his emotional state was always really unpredictable.

When Dad and I went to restaurants, he would order a drink and start dancing in a booth, on top of the chair, then attempt to get on top of the table before the manager came over to settle him down. It was beyond embarrassing for a teenager who had acquaintances from school who worked at these fine establishments. Luckily, most of my friends just thought he was "mad cool," but I was always on edge because I knew the possibility of him switching the other way to angry and violent could happen on a drop of a dime.

I spent my days waiting for that dime to drop. It was when my older half-sister, Dad's daughter from a previous relationship, and her friends came to visit. We didn't have much of a relationship except for occasional weekend visits when they came to get Dad to buy them booze and party. This was their first visit since Dad admitted he had a problem, but he didn't tell them. I felt really uneasy. I told Dad I wasn't sure if him buying them booze was a good idea. He said, "I'm fine, hun. Just relax and be cool." I hated when he said that to me. I had a strong sense that things were about to fall apart so it was extremely hard for me to just "be cool."

Early in the evening, a few of my guy friends stopped by to check out my sister and her friends who were partying at my house. Thankfully they were somewhat unimpressed and left early. My best friend Gabby was there with me. I felt safe with her; I needed someone on my side who knew what was going on. Gabby knew just enough about my dad's ping pong of relapses and recovery, but she did not know about the unpredictable possible scenarios that could play out. We watched my sister and her friends get intoxicated. Dad seemed to be okay, but then he started drinking. I got nervous. He was pacing a lot, getting really energized in a way that seemed like he was agitated and needed something.

The phone rang and I ran to get it in case it was Dwayne, his dealer. Dad got it before me. I grabbed it out of his hands and screamed, "Dad! No! Don't do it!" I snapped. I had never been so bold as to stand up to Dad before that moment, but I felt that his life depended on it. In a blink of an eye, he threw the phone at me, then threw me into the stairs, grabbed me by the arms, shook me violently, got right in my face and said, "Don't you *EVER* do that again!" He thrust me into the stairs again and left. He got in his car and peeled out of the driveway. One of my sister's friends managed to jump into the car with him and my sister followed them in her car. I don't know what happened afterward except that Gabby and I ended up at her house. That night I began to tell her bits and pieces about what was going on.

The next day when I got back home, my sister and her friends told me their versions of what happened the rest of the night. Dad was nowhere to be found. They shared their stories as if they were in an exciting scene in a movie. But this was reality, my actual life. I was disgusted because they would just have "crazy wild stories" to tell back in little bumble town Pennsylvania while I stayed behind cleaning up the pieces of what my life had become living with Dad. It was a double life somewhere between hell and high school.

A few months later and many sleepless nights without Dad at home, I was getting closer to wanting to make a big change in my life. I could not handle having the burden of being his only family anymore. My body felt the weight of it all. No one was looking out for me, not even me. I was being neglected and there was no sign that Dad was going to get back on the path of recovery in a serious manner. It was time to step in and put on my oxygen mask before this plane crashed and burned.

The Escape

By the end of February, I decided it was time to leave. I had to do something different or else I would soon be driven to insanity. It had been at least three or four times that Dad didn't come home on a weeknight; I began calling Mom to let her in on more of what was going on. The last time was the evening of one of my dance performances, which came and went. There was no sign of Dad who was supposed to be there to watch me perform and drive me home. I had taken two buses to get to my performance early for rehearsal before the show. After waiting for over an hour after my show, I somehow managed to get a ride home with a friend's parent. I went to bed, still no Dad.

The next morning, he still was not home, so I called Mom. She was furious. We went to lunch to talk things over. She said she wanted me out of that house no matter how devoted I was to Dad. For the first time in my life, I agreed with her. I was done and ready for a new life. Where would it be though? My mom said jokingly, "Well, you can always go live with Gramma in Texas for a little while." That was it. It was exactly what I had to do. I needed to escape. I needed to go far away from my crumbling life and Gramma was a safe place.

The next few days were a blur as we made plans to get me to my new home in Texas, my new beginning. Mom bought my plane ticket, arranged my school records to be transferred, and I said my goodbyes to friends without any real explanation as to why I was leaving. The whole time I was completely numb; at least until that last night when I went back to tell Dad.

When we got there, he was with some drugged-out woman I had never seen before. They were both extremely high. His eyes were bright red. Mom took Dad upstairs to his bedroom and reprimanded him like a little boy. He took it just like that as he sat there avoiding eye contact with her, looking at the ground, nodding his head saying, "I know. You're right, Brenda." Mom scolded him by saying things like, "What the hell are you doing with your life, Jay? You are going to get AIDS! You are going to get yourself killed. You are not being a good father to your daughter like you promised you would."

As I eavesdropped from my room while I packed, I realized that Dad had begged Mom to keep me when she left him. He believed, and perhaps she believed too, that I was the only reason he would survive. I gave him purpose and a reason to wake up in the morning. When he begged her, seven years prior, he promised that he would take care of me and make it his purpose to be my father.

By the time I was ready to leave and Mom was loading up the car with my stuff, Dad was on the couch downstairs and the crackhead woman was gone. I walked downstairs apprehensively, to say my last goodbye. It was going to be the last time I would see Dad for a very long time; we both knew it but didn't speak of it. He said nothing to me at all. He felt like a ghost. His hair was wild, his bloodshot eyes were vacant, he was a shell of a body, and his soul was no longer in there. He was no longer my daddy.

I announced it was time for me to go. No response. I said how sorry I was for leaving him. He couldn't even look at me when he got up and walked me to the front door. I followed. There were heavy tears in my eyes waiting to escape but I was trying my best to be strong. When I got to the door, I tried to hug him for a moment and then he pushed me away. He pushed me out the door like I was a stranger invading his space. He pushed me outside and shut the door. My daddy was gone, and I felt like it was somehow my fault.

I slowly walked through the downpour to Mom's car, doing my best to remain strong. I sat in the car, shut the door, and immediately years of tears that I had never shed exploded from my body. I sat there crying for a very long time, for what felt like days; I am still there in some ways.

Mom just sat there watching me, her only daughter, her little girl, crying and falling apart. There was nothing she could do but just be a witness. I fogged up the windows with my sobs and tears. She didn't say anything. She couldn't. She just sat there. What else could she do? Her little girl was broken and from just that simple knowing, she was severely broken too.

She probably thought back to all the moments years before when she considered sneaking out in the middle of the night and leaving with her baby bundled up to never look back. She probably thought about it and regretted the time she finally did leave but left her daughter behind instead. She must have known somehow this was meant to be, at least I like to believe this to be true. She knew that I had to learn who my dad really was, the beautiful soul she once fell in love with back when they first met in that town in Pennsylvania with the lion years ago. She knew that the stories would have never done him justice. No, Mom knew I had to know for myself, even with the pain and suffering that was there at our doorstep on that dreadful night. She watched me weep with such sorrow, a sorrow that would permeate both of our souls and haunt us for years. This wound was deep and primal for me. It was a wound that I would have to sleep with and keep there in my dreams for years because it hurt way too much to bring it out to the light to heal. It would take the miracle of Dad dying for that process to begin.

ACT TWO

DARK DANCES OF THE SOUL

The dark night of the soul comes just before
revelation. When everything is lost, and all seems darkness,
then comes the new life and all that is needed.

— *Joseph Campbell*

Letter to Radiant One

Dear Radiant One,

We are entering now into the story where I wrestle with my shadows and make friends with them in some way. As we dive in more deeply, you may begin to see how the stories of my childhood molded some patterns and stories of my adulthood. We will find our way through my darkness as I dance with my emotions. Pay attention to how your body speaks to you as I share how I detangled myself from some of the patterns and accepted other pieces of them. You may begin to also unpack your own experiences with the somatic and expanded awareness practices that helped me (and continue to help me) along my path. I hope they can be of service through your own emotional recovery and healing.

When I first began to write this book, it was like a healing for me, and as the many layers unfolded, I realized how it can be deep healing for all of us if we choose to lean in. Even if you do not feel that you need it now, I hope you lean in because there might be something unexpected for you. Those moments you feel the resistance in the shadows of grief, fear, anger, shame, loneliness, anxiety, and numbness, I encourage you to lean in. Your soul found the way to this book, but your ego might resist the transformation that may begin to occur as you go. That is okay, it just wants to keep you comfortable in your discomfort. Trust these resources are here for you when you are ready. Come to them when they call you and see what happens.

With grace,

Phoebe

Letter to Grief

Dear Grief,

As I write this, you are sitting quite close to me. I lost another loved one this week. Gabby was my best friend who was in my life since first grade when we bonded over our white stockings with red hearts on the school playground. She was such a fashionista even back then. We became best friends in third grade when we were in Mrs. Smith's class together, and realized we lived just half a block away from each other. That was the school year when I needed a friend most after my parents split up. She was a constant in terms of the love we had for each other, even though we fluttered in and out of each other's lives over time. I knew even when she was grounded by her parents, a bribe with Pringles would get her to escape and come to my home. We would listen to music and dance together, and as adults, she was always a phone call away even in the middle of the night when I felt alone. I loved her like a sister, unconditionally.

I can't even really begin to explain the relationship that I had with this soul or how I am feeling now knowing she is no longer of this world. But having to go through this process with you again, Grief, I think I am beginning to understand you a bit better. Grief, what I know of you is you hold everything in the experience of you: depression, numbness, joy, laughter, anger, guilt, gratitude, fear, acceptance. All of it.

You shook me to my core when I lost my dad the second time when he officially left his body. These last eight years, I have somehow felt his presence and support in ways that I never felt before when he was on this Earth. Because of that, I feel way more at peace about Gabs. Even though it makes no sense at all that she at age forty-three, my age, is now gone, having died in her sleep from a potentially treatable autoimmune disease. It is strange as I write this; I weirdly sensed this unfolding of events, just as I did unconsciously months before the passing of my dad.

Over this year I allowed some relationships to shed, while others flourished. Gabs and I didn't reach out much this past year. In fact, our last exchange was when the lockdown was unfolding and I was still in Bali, and she told me to be safe as I traveled back. I wrote to her one other time with a picture of a few high school friends I reconnected with, but she never responded. That all felt okay though. I felt good knowing she was in Morocco, safe and happy. From what I could tell, she was in a good place.

These past two weeks, she was on my mind as I wrote some of the stories on these pages. She always seemed to be in the background of most of them, and she was always a friend I could count on in those moments. The only one who held my secrets for no one else to know. She was an angel in some ways. Just a few days ago, I felt called to look back at a period in my life when I was in college and saw how the choices I made back then really set the stage of my adult life. I have been experiencing time in such a different way recently and have reflected on the characters of my story. What did they each represent?

Gabby came to mind and there was a huge unfolding of memories, feelings, shadows, light, music, dance, and so much more. I was overwhelmed and decided to set it all aside thinking we would talk in a few days on my birthday. I figured that we would have a good long talk then and I would tell her about the journey of writing this book and how she played such a big role in my life. But that day did not come as I had envisioned. We only talk through her spirit now. She is no longer in her pain body, she is free and now back to being formless, back to the stars as she has always intended to be.

Gabby struggled with her body image since we were kids and the mysterious pain, sleeping disorder, and inexplicable weight loss over her last nine years seemed to haunt her. I sometimes think now that she just had too much damn energy for her body to hold it all in. She needed to be free, to be with her mom again. As I sit here now, on Easter after three days of crying, laughing, dancing, and feeling anger and joy all wrapped together, I know this is how it has to be.

Grief, through these last eight years, you have taught me well about non-attachment as I made my own emotional recovery. You have taught me to feel in a way I avoided for most of my life. I am grateful for you and the lessons you brought me. As you come to my doorstep again with the departure of my best friend, I even see how she was the perfect person to show me the growth I have endured. Gabby was never mine to claim, she belonged to everyone whose presence she graced. We fluttered in and out of each other's lives over the years. We never really ran in the same circles, but we always knew where and how to find each other when needed.

I can sit here and feel guilty for not communicating more these last two years but we both know better than that now. Gramma said something about you when the news came in about Gabs. She said, "Your Grief will turn into something good. It always does. Trust that."

I will never invite you in but know when you enter my home, I will welcome you with open arms. I will ask you, what do you bring me with this package wrapped up in sorrow? And I will know whatever it is, it all belongs.

With grace,

Phoebe

Grief Has No Rules

The story I intended to write on this subject matter now has a whole other layer to it because of this recent loss.

Part of the story begins in the summer of 2012. I had a new job as a director of yoga at a boutique hotel in the Hudson Valley. I had the freedom to create this program from the ground up. My whole life was finally clicking into place. Married to my college boyfriend, John, we moved into our first home as homeowners earlier that spring, and not just any home, my dream home. John was nervous about our finances when we bought the house since my steady salary was not yet guaranteed but I said, "just trust." I knew in my bones I was getting this gig and I did just a few months later. My dad was back in my life and sober too. We enjoyed having him come for visits to our new home.

In August, just before my yoga program opened in September, I got a bad cold. I was feeling the pressure of my new job and John was not helping. Things were tense when his family came to visit. My dad had come to visit us one of the days to see John's family (his dad and my dad had the special connection of being Vietnam vets). Even though I wasn't feeling great during the family visit, I lit up when Dad was around. I always did. Since he entered back in my life a few years earlier, I wanted to make the most of every little moment we had together. John seemed annoyed by this and picked a fight with me when I said the next morning that I was feeling sick again and needed to rest. The rest of the morning, I stayed in my bedroom crying. His mom even pulled me aside and asked if he was being abusive to me.

After his family left, we went to see a minor league baseball game across the river at Duchess Stadium. While we were waiting in line to buy tickets, we ran into one of his coworkers and her boyfriend. At some point, John insisted we go sit with them for a bit to break up the tension the two were experiencing—they were fighting or amid a breakup. I thought it was a little weird that John would know that about his coworker, who was much younger than us, and that he felt obligated to sit with them because of it. It was a passing thought, and I didn't get too invested in it.

At the end of the game there were fireworks, the only real reason I enjoyed going to the game. The coworker's boyfriend worked at the fire department and was responsible for letting them off, so they excused themselves when that time came. John and I stayed to watch the spectacular light show. There was smoke, a lot of smoke. There was so much smoke that I started to cough; I could not breathe. Between my cold and the smoke, I felt like I was having an asthma attack, but I didn't have asthma. I covered my face with my shirt to filter out the smoke. It didn't help; I kept coughing and gasping for air. People looked at me in horror. I could not tell if they felt helpless and wanted to try to help me or were completely annoyed and inconvenienced by my lack of breathing. It continued as we took the long walk back to the car. When I got in the car, I did what Dad had always told me to do when I cried to a point of anxiety and hyperventilation, I put my head between my legs. My lungs were on fire, and I felt them as they contracted with a burning sensation that was suffocating me. The air was pure toxicity. John asked if I wanted to go to the hospital. That made me even more anxious. I kept trying to take in a breath of fresh air, but it felt like a trap door was locking any air in and keeping any new air out.

Finally, when we crossed the bridge back to our home, I found some composure. My chest felt extremely heavy, but my breath returned with a little ease. I lay in bed with John and felt the weight in my chest as it still struggled to rise and fall, carrying a new wispy sound. Despite what I had just gone through, I needed to have sex with John. It had been way too long, and I felt it had to be then. As I initiated, he asked, "Are you sure?" I don't know what possessed me at that moment, but I felt it was my only choice to feel better; it was as if somehow everything depended on it.

The asthma-like attack turned into full-blown bronchitis. For the next four months, I visited doctors and specialists and tried various inhalers and steroids to kick it. Finally, I went to a specialist to breathe in a high dose of steroids in a small, boxed room. My lungs finally started to feel some relief by December.

During that time, I opened the yoga program with much success, working long hours and spending little time at home, and didn't see Dad at all. By the time I was feeling a bit better in early December, Dad came to visit me for a Daddy/Daughter Day. Just the two of us. We went for lunch at one of my favorite places and got a quiche. He bought a whole quiche to take home. (He freakin' loved his quiche.) I took him to my new job to show him my yoga studio that overlooked the waterfall and mountain. He was rather quiet, and I wondered what was on his mind. He said how proud he was of me, but I felt there was something else that he wanted to say. He got like that sometimes, super quiet, like he felt something that wasn't there yet. He seemed to have more of those moments now that he was sober and rehabilitated.

I saw him one more time at Christmas—our first Christmas together since I was fourteen years old and, unbeknownst to us, our last. My whole family was there: Dad, Mom, my younger half-sister, John, and me. What more could I have asked for? It was all coming together after a very long and winding road, we made it home, to my home.

I will never forget our last moments together that Christmas day. Dad and I stood in my doorway while everyone else lounged in the dining room around the food. We hugged each other: a big, long hug, like we always did since our reunion. It was much different from the time we said a final goodbye when he pushed me out of my home at fourteen on that very rainy night. This time, as we said goodbye, we took our time and looked into each other's eyes. He said, "I love you, hun" and I replied enthusiastically like a little kid, "I love you, DAD!" As I look back now, I hear the voices and laughter dimly in the background, yet this moment with my dad is in full focus, everything else blurry. He walked out of the door into his little Porsche Boxster that in less than a month I would inherit. I yelled at him to text me when he got home. I continued to stand in the doorway as he started the car and prepared for his journey: set up his music, turned on his GPS, lit a cigarette, put his riding gloves on, and then, just like that he drove out of my driveway and out of my life for the last time.

Two weeks later, on January 9th, 2013, I got a call from the New Haven Police Department while I was at work. My dad was dead. He died from a heart attack in his sleep the night before.

The next two months after my dad died, Grief and I were super tight. It seeped into my life and took over at moments that were not appropriate, like teaching my yoga class or sitting in a meeting with my coworkers. It got to a point where I had to sit down and negotiate when I could spend time with Grief. Friday was my preferred time to be alone when I did not have to work. On Fridays, I gave Grief a permission slip to run the show. It could make me cry, scream out loud, tear things apart, look at old photo albums, call a friend to cry to or laugh with, get lost in music and dance, or watch movies that made me feel joy or sadness or all of it. Sometimes Grief was about feeling numb and making a fire and watching it all day. Whatever bag of weird wanted to come out was welcome in the safety and privacy of my home.

John knew this and his Fridays in the city started to get longer and longer. I would try my best to wrap up my crying and grieving by the time he got home, but there was no guarantee with Grief once I let the little freak out of the bag. I didn't quite know the rules around Grief or what to expect. You see, this was the first time I allowed myself to grieve. When I left my dad and then he disappeared, there was literally no space to grieve. I did not tell any of my friends the truth about my dad, except Gabby, and my family did not talk too much about it. It crept into the crevices of my life in bouts that were inexplicable to myself and others over the rest of my early adulthood. It would sneak in with outbursts of crying from dreams or hysterical breakdowns when John or other ex-boyfriends would leave me, and I feared I would never see them again. I didn't know that Grief had its own rules, meaning there are no rules and it carried everything— sadness, rage, denial, joy, gratitude, heaviness, and confusion. You probably have read the textbooks too and maybe even felt it at this point in your life. Bottom line, I was unraveling with Grief.

By March, it was still heavy for me. The first Friday of March was another late-night cry session. It had been cold, dreary, and snowing all day which gave me a permission slip to get really dark and twisty. By the time John got home late that evening, I was still in it. He watched me curled up on a couch balled up as a big wet, sobbing mess. He just sat there watching from the other side of the room, on another couch; he watched me weep for my daddy and did nothing. I could not say anything but in my mind, I was screaming at him, *Come sit next to me!! Hold me!!!! I feel so utterly alone!* He never got that message. I wept myself to sleep.

The very next morning, I woke up to the sun beaming on my face, eagerly asking me to see the new day that it was giving me. I looked at my phone: 75 degrees and Abundant Sunshine. A breath of fresh freakin' air!!! I got up to teach with a pep in my step that I had not felt in months, maybe even a year! On my drive back home after class, I had big plans to celebrate the new day with John. I brought us back a nice spread of food for lunch intending to take a picnic and go for a hike. Grief let go of its grip on this day and I wanted us to celebrate!

But then, in a blink of an eye, the clouds rolled through, and it was there again with a new friend, Betrayal. John wanted a divorce. My heart sank and I watched all the possibilities of being happy again speed away from me, leaving me behind in a dark, abandoned well of despair.

None of it made sense at that moment (but looking it back now, I don't know how I could not have seen it coming). We talked for hours about his mental health, his admission to still abusing drugs without my knowledge, and how all that was wrapped up in him not wanting to be married anymore. The next day we took our hike and talked some more. I tried to make sense of it all. As we spoke, I felt like we had been living two separate lives under the same roof for the last several years and I was just becoming aware of it. Within a day's time, it felt like I didn't know this person, my husband, anymore. I took a selfie of us on that hike and when I look back at it, I can see the deadness in his eyes, his soul dim, and the desperation in mine.

For the next several months, I grieved for both the loss of my dad and my marriage, a fifteen-year relationship. During that time, I found my way to an acupuncturist to help me with a few issues I was having. I filled out the very long form asking me every little symptom, illness, and injury I had in the last ten years. When it came to lungs, I checked off bronchitis. After speaking with me about my current lifestyle changes and what was happening in my life, she reviewed my form. She looked at me over the paper and asked when I had bronchitis. I replied, "Last summer and fall, why?" Her eyes softened and she put her hand on my hand and she said, "My dear, you have been grieving way before this all happened. Your body knew before you did." As I quickly learned from her, in Chinese medicine the organ that carries the energy of grief is the lungs. I then flashed back to the night of the fireworks and that coworker, *the girl* as I now called her.

As the detangling from my marriage continued, it was also revealed that John was engaging inappropriately with that coworker from the fireworks night. Somehow my body knew. No wonder it was on fire with Grief and begged for sex in an attempt to save the marriage that night. It knew my marriage was doomed. Grief is a wise one.

Now, the added layer here is Gabby. During that same summer of doom, Gabby was having problems of her own. She had been working in the nightlife world for many years as a manager of a club in SoHo, and her body was also talking to her then. She wasn't well. Her body was breaking down and emotionally, she was breaking down too. She was coming up to visit me on her weekends to recover from the stress. She would mostly just sleep all day and night in my yoga room with little respites to come to chat with me, eat, and sit in our sauna. She was scared. Her mom, Olivia, died of breast cancer when we were in high school, and Gabby felt like she might be doomed like her mom. Olivia was beautiful and somewhat iconic in both of our eyes, and her light burned out way too soon. Gabby's fears eventually came true nine years later when she received the diagnosis that ended her days on this Earth.

I still don't know how to make sense of it fully, but somehow her passing reflects this journey of sharing these stories with you. Gabby is interwoven throughout my life and most of these stories. As I grieve for her, I grieve the past that I carried for so long, a burden that I can no longer carry with me. These stories are now released on these pages for you to digest, learn, and grow from.

At the end of this section, I will ask you a few questions for when you have to sit with Grief.

One question is, what does this person or situation you grieve represent to you? For me, Gabby represents so much joy, freedom, confidence, strength, resiliency, elegance, laughter, music, dance, and light. Many people who knew Gabby could easily see she was a bright starlight; you could not deny experiencing her when she shined.

But Gabby also represents sorrow, heaviness, insecurity, fragility, illness, anger, and darkness, for reasons I will not divulge for they are her stories to tell in some other form now. It is safe to share my side of things though. Gabs held my hand through some dark moments of my life: when I drank for the first time and saw myself as my dad, when he disappeared, through various fights with John over the years, when I went through the loss of my dad again, and through my divorce. Gabby was there. She reflected my fragile insecurities about my outer beauty when she seemed flawless on the outside, and yet only I knew she was crumbling on the inside. I was sometimes jealous that she could hide it so well with a stunning outfit, a good camera angle, or a mood-altering playlist. I never uttered these words to her but as I write this, I can hear her say to me, "Aw! Phoeeeebes! You are so beautiful, and I am in awe and inspired by you too!"

So, what am I ready to release with Gabby? I am ready to release these absurd thoughts that I wasn't good enough or cool enough. I free myself from the weight we both carried from the loss of our parents, the traumas we both endured, and the chaos we both searched out in our own ways.

What do I want to embody to carry on her spirit? I want to embody her love and passion for music and dance. I will carry on her grace, her fierceness, and her love for beautiful things. Somehow, she thought I was one of them, so I will embrace her spirit through my beauty.

It All Belongs in Grief

This is the simplest emotion which we can more or less identify in time and space after an event of loss occurs. Yet, grief is the most complex because it holds everything and has no distinct timeline. With other emotions, like anger or joy, there is an arc of energy. There is something that triggers it; you feel it in your body and once it is given some kind of expression, there is usually some decline of the initial heightened state. With grief, it holds all the emotions, and they are all over the map with no real order. Sure, you can

Google grief and see all the steps that take you to end at the gates of Acceptance. It's not that perfect though.

If grief was a shape, it would be a spiral. There might be small moments where you turn the corner at acceptance but then something triggers you. The next moment you can feel angry that your loved one is gone, or you feel guilty for something you said or didn't say, or you have a moment you forget they are even gone or start crying again in a puddle of photos. Just know, it all belongs. And if you get on the road that ends at the Gates of Acceptance, you might also wind up back on Blues Alley or Angry Birds Court, or whatever it might be for you in that time/space.

It. All. Belongs.

It doesn't matter how long it takes you. You might grieve for your dad a week but your dog for two years; it's all okay. Sometimes it gets easier and sometimes it doesn't and you have to start all over again.

It's all okay.

I will say that if you add more healthy resources like the following to your grieving toolbox, the process of grief may flow through you a bit easier. Before we get there, let's talk about grief energetically in the body.

Grief At the Heart of It

As I mentioned in my story, in Chinese medicine, grief is expressed in the lungs. I will not dive more deeply into that since that is not my place of expertise, but I will touch on the subtle body energy system, the chakra system which we observe in yoga, and other Eastern teachings. In this system, we look at energy throughout our body as wheels or discs, spinning to keep us in a balanced flow state where too much or too little will bring our energy out of balance. Like the meridians in Chinese medicine, the lung and heart area is where we feel and express our grief; this wheel of energy we call the heart chakra. It is the home of our heart and lungs and can also be expressed out into the arms and hands.

When we are in balance, we feel loved, connected, and more compassionate within ourselves and with our outer world. When we are out of balance in the heart chakra, we can feel unloved, disconnected, or shielded from the outer world. What can trigger this imbalance is grief which will be our main focus in the practices shortly.

In our Western world, we also speak of grief through the body. When we experience a loss, we say we have a "heavy heart" or that we are "heartbroken." When we are depressed and heartbroken, we tend to carry ourselves with a collapsed chest to unconsciously protect our vulnerable hearts and close ourselves off from the outer world. We sit crouched over the rest of the body, only take in a certain amount of life force energy (our breath) into our lungs, and collapse on the diaphragm, which makes our breath short and hollow. We don't allow ourselves to take in any more life for the sake of losing it again.

Think about the attack in my lungs during those fireworks: It expressed itself as an asthma attack on my lungs, but it was really, on a much deeper level, the attack on my marriage. I violently felt it in my body and fought it by insisting on making love that night.

Your body knows and it wants you to listen.

As you read this, how do you feel in your heart space? Are you catching yourself in the posture that I just identified and now adjusting yourself? Think back to other moments you felt *off* in this heart and lung space, did you have a string of chest colds that you couldn't kick, a heart attack, heartburn, an arm or shoulder injury? Do you remember what else was going on in your life that your body was maybe trying to express? Just allow yourself to sit with this a bit and ponder if there was a deeper message for you. Were you not feeling the love and connection you needed in some way from yourself or from others at that time? Just listen and feel what comes up. Maybe it is time for you to see it and understand it for what it is.

I remember during my grieving, I came into a restorative backbend, a place that had usually felt safe and very comfortable for me to rest. On this day, I couldn't do it without tears flowing and a sharp stabbing feeling under my right shoulder blade. It didn't feel safe to open my heart again because I felt like I was getting stabbed in my back by the person I loved, a man who I was married to who abandoned me after the loss of another man, my dad. Something also to note, the right side of the body energetically is our masculine side, and the left side of our body is our feminine energetic side. When we begin to think of our bodies as maps to our story, we begin to see how beautifully poetic and real it is communicating with us. In my mid-twenties I was on the cusp of making big life decisions to leave my path of dance and to get married. During this time, my left (feminine side) hip was in so much pain, so much so that I thought I would need a hip replacement before I was thirty. My hip echoed my fears of taking the next steps forward into the unknown spaces of life. Once I made the choices and stepped forward with action, the pain went away.

These are just some examples of how we can start to decode our bodies. There are many books out there that can help you; one of my personal favorites is *You Can Heal Your*

Life by Louise Hay. What I think is most important to remember though is you are the storyteller of your body, the one who holds the key to decoding what it wants to say.

Let's Check In

First, honor whatever emotion is present. It might be heart-wrenching snotty, sobs of sadness to hysterical laughter where you feel you might pee yourself and everything in between. Welcome all of it. Be with all of it. Find people who feel safe and allow all of this to flow through you. Some of the feelings may surprise you.

Honor what is present. If you don't know, ask Grief.

Ask Grief, "What do you think I am ready to experience today?" And just listen.

Then, give it expression. Go through the steps for anger, sadness, shame, guilt, or fear, all of which I cover here.

Don't clamp down on it! Let it flow through you. The more you resist it, the more it will bottle up and explode when you can least control it. Trust the process.

One of the practices I found especially helpful for connecting with my grief was a writing meditation. If you are feeling stuck in your grief, try this for yourself. Once there is a little space from the initial shock of your loss, sit quietly with a journal and pen. Maybe do a little bit of movement and meditation. Light candles, incense, sage, palo santo, your lost one's favorite cigarettes, or whatever you feel called to light. Put on an article of their clothing or an outfit you wore when spending a special day with them. Have their letters, pictures, or mementos out on a little altar to honor them. Do whatever feels good to get into a space where you can invite their spirit in and have a conversation.

Then, write them a letter. Don't hold back. Again, let it flow.

If it feels right, let your hand receive the words from them to write you a letter back.

Release it through a ceremony. Burn it somewhere safe to send into the ether and to the spirit world.

Now, answer the following journal questions and keep them.

- What does this person or situation that is no longer in my life represent for me?

- Is there something I can release with her/him/them/it?

- Is there something I can celebrate and be a vessel for the energy she/he/them/it represents?

- How can I commit to this to honor her/him/them/it?

Sit with your response for a bit and allow whatever feels good to come with you into your day. Notice as you write how your body responds to the words that you choose.

Now, whatever you are feeling in this moment, finish this statement:

Grief wants me to experience the story of...

Letter to Fear and Abandonment

Dear Fear,

You kept me from doing some amazing things in my life. You have always known how to play your cards with me; I create a bond with someone and then you take them away from me in an instant. Fear of Abandonment, that's your full name to me.

I saw Abandonment in all its forms as a child: physical, mental, emotional, spiritual. Mom left me alone with Dad. He left me in all ways through his flashbacks, his drug use, and then his actual disappearance for sixteen years. I felt abandoned by the Universe during these times, with no one to listen, see, or support me.

In 2013, Abandonment stripped everything away from me: my dad, my husband, my home, my pets, my health, my stability, my safety, my trust in people and myself. It left me feeling hollow and depleted from my heart being ripped out of my body. Fear, you lingered after Abandonment destroyed my life and you convinced me everyone was a threat, everyone would leave me, and I would always have to fend for myself. You triggered the feeling that my heart could be ripped out again, whenever anyone got close. I felt my tethered little heart, pulsating with you while trying to be strong to anchor within me. The thing is, I figured you both out. I am on the path to building my home within myself now, so that when anyone is taken away again, I know I will be okay.

I had a vision recently of my young self. She was sitting, curled up in a ball looking outward with a deep heaviness in her heart because as she looked out, she didn't see anyone looking back at her. I was there though. I was carrying a torch for her and circling around her, to make sure the outer world would not harm her anymore. Then, I heard a voice tell me to turn towards her. I put down the torch, turned around, saw her, and held her in my arms. I told her everything was okay. She cried joyful tears because she finally felt held, heard, and seen. We both felt the warmth of our embrace. You see, my back to her was for protection the whole time, but she didn't know this. She only saw a back to her, a back to her was still abandonment. She knows that I am here now, and I will never let her go. We will dance, play, bring joy and radiance into our world together.

Your scary scenarios of people leaving us have no power over us anymore.

You also convinced me to be afraid of my own gifts of feeling and sensing both my inner and outer worlds. Fear, you made me believe that I created the scenes that played out in my life, like the times I felt the energy change with Dad just moments before he went into a rage and hurt people that I was mad at. You convinced me I was cursed because of this ability to feel things. I buried this curse of mine, at least I tried to, so that I didn't have to face it all again, but it somehow made you stronger. It made me scared that it might happen again at any moment, without a warning if I thought something that might hurt someone. You have been so intertwined in my life for so long.

I am grateful though, that you kept me away from danger during these times. There were so many times in my life where things could have gone horribly wrong, and you were there to protect me. But to convince me afterward that I was the one who created these scenarios, and to tell me I was still in danger, that I was never safe from my thoughts even when I was alone, that was wrong of you.

Summing up what Elizabeth Gilbert says, Fear, you can be in the backseat to let me know when there is something to avoid, only when necessary, but you cannot be in the driver's seat. You can't ride shotgun either to play with the temperature controls to determine how I feel or radio controls to determine what I listen to.

I embrace my gifts now. I see their worth and my worth because of them. Thank you for your service but you will take the backseat. I am grateful we could have this conversation.

With love,

Phoebe

Seeds of Fear

Abandonment. I think this is a wound many feel on some level, no matter how loved we were by our parents. For my story, it was and has been a very confusing one. Both of my parents abandoned me in their ways, but also really loved me in a special way that I always knew was there, even in those darker moments. The night my parents split up, I watched the fireflies fly up, and my whole life as I knew it imploded. In the background, I still heard my parents fighting over who was going to get Phoebe. My mom loved me, and she needed to leave my dad *and* she also knew I needed to stay with him, to give him a purpose. My dad loved me, even when he locked me out that horrible night and I cried for him to let me in. All the other times he pushed me out of the way, it felt like he was somehow protecting me from himself and from the demons that resided within him. I felt it even when he pushed me out the door without a hug or a goodbye that rainy night, and then I sat in the car waiting for Mom to hold me. All those moments I felt so alone as a child, yet I felt loved. It made all my relationships confusing. I could not hold bonds with friends or in intimate relationships because even though I felt loved, with no evidence, I believed that they would leave me, so I pushed them away before that day would come.

It wasn't until I got married that I started to believe that someone would stay with me and love me unconditionally. I gave everything to that relationship—he did too for a while. But at some point, we entered the pattern of abandonment again, with his drug use and eventually calling it all off. After eight years of recovery from that devastating year of loss, I am just now feeling like I can trust myself again; I no longer always have the voice of Fear in my ear.

What shifted? Eight years of grueling work, showing up for myself day after day. I had to build trust in my choices again, in the people I surrounded myself with, and how I chose to be there for myself lovingly and gently. When I had the vision just recently of my young self who wanted me to just hold her, I think that was the real moment it all clicked. But it came from a lot of courageous work, of standing up for myself and sending people away who didn't show up reciprocally. The most recent step, the pandemic, grounded me in one place to be with myself with no escape or distraction.

Fear of my gifts. I remember first sensing my gifts as a very young child that moment with the bulldog cornering me in my kitchen. Our eyes met and I felt some kind of pain or anxious energy behind those big brown eyes. I remember not understanding why he was so mad or why I was there in front of him, but I sensed that memory was important, like some kind of blueprint for my life.

I remember lying in bed as a child trying to go as far back as I could in my memory, and I always landing there. It is a mystery why the significance of dogs has played out in my life and embedded into my body as was revealed in that healing session at the beginning of this book. Why did these dogs represent fear at pivotal moments in my life? As a child, I was afraid of so much, but never really of dogs. I was aware of their power and ferocity, but it never got in the way of being me with them.

I recall the Doberman we had for only a couple of weeks when I was six. I clearly remember sitting in a chair in the breeder's office, my parents being interviewed by the breeder. Looking at the photos of other Dobermans they had bred and their various certificates, ribbons, and all the other brag-worthy things that hang on breeders' walls, I neither felt fear nor worry.

The next memory I have is the dog being at home with us. He was big, and a bit scary when it came to people coming to our door. I don't remember him really caring much about me. I was just a little body that ran around the house, and I didn't really care much about him, except when someone came to our door, and he barked a ferocious bark. He only lasted a few weeks in our house when Mom decided he was too threatening to visitors at our door, specifically my aunt who was staying with us, and the postman. I can still see his silhouette at the door: Big, tall, and regal, with a dark, smooth coat, pointy ears, and his mouth slightly opened to prepare for a bark attack at the door.

I have a clear vision of my aunt walking up the sidewalk and this dog jumping on his hind legs at the door to lunge at her. I remember feeling a moment of tension in my body. I stood to attention and made a conscious choice not to let this dog ever know I was scared. So, with that thought, I quickly shook off the tension and went back to playing as if he wasn't even there.

There was Saatchi, my Akita, who was one of my best friends and protectors. So many times, when I feared what Dad might do, she was there by my side keeping him in check; she was always ready to nip him in the ass if he came too close to me in a way that might threaten us. When Saatchi was nearby, my body always felt safe. She was at least twenty pounds heavier than me, and I always felt like she knew it was her job to keep me relaxed, loved, and protected.

Then there was my dog, Newks. I sensed things with him that I was too scared to face until it was too late. We got him during an unstable time in my marriage. While John was dealing with knee surgery, a drug addiction, and being diagnosed with a mental illness, we decided to get a puppy. He came into our New York City home before the holidays and brutal winter, while my husband walked with a cane, while I worked several jobs all over the city most days and was never home to properly walk a pup. We talked about all the obstacles we had against having a dog and we still did it, with the agreement that we were both all in.

Life lesson: Don't make an agreement that could possibly be a crazy one with someone who is dealing with a mental illness and when you are questioning your own mental wellness too. We had Newks for a week and I came home to the adoption contract on the table. John was done. I sat him down and explained we had an agreement that we were all in and that for the puppy's own sake, we had to commit to keeping him. He had already been in a home and foster care for three months; it was our responsibility to provide a stable home. The irony, right? Somehow, we thought our chaotic life would provide stability for all of us. The equation did not quite add up in this case.

Newks was a challenge for us. He quickly decided who was cool to come into our place and who wasn't. Luckily, we agreed with him in most cases, and with the ones we didn't, we tried our best to work around it. The hardest part was walking this cute pup in the city when everyone and their baby wanted to stop and pet him. He was cute and fluffy and had a look as if he was ready to play but he could turn on a dime.

One day we were outside of our building, about to get in a quick walk before I had to run to teach. We ran into a neighbor and her daughter. The mother could talk for a long time, and I didn't have the time that day. I said my pleasantries and tried to get on my way. She kept talking. Her daughter was taunting Newks; I gave him a little tug to sit so he would not get riled up. The daughter kept waving her hands in his face, while the mother kept talking and ignoring my comments about "having to run." I felt the tension in my body rising, my heart beating. My eyes darted between the mother, the daughter, my dog. I felt it a split second before it happened, Newkie's mouth dug into the little face of the girl. I got my hand in there and pried her free. She was crying and bleeding. I reprimanded my dog and tended to make sure the little girl was okay. The mom apologized to me that her girl was too rambunctious, and I said, "Oh my! No! I am so sorry! This should have never happened! I can't believe he did this! What can I do?" She took her daughter into her apartment. The adrenaline pulsed through my body, I took my dog quickly to finish the walk and he just pranced down the street as if nothing happened. I called John and he went to the neighbor to see if he could help in any way. The little girl ended up needing a few stitches and the mom never pressed charges or reported Newks. Instead, she took the blame. I was so very hurt and ashamed to have a pet so vicious, but mostly because *I felt it*. I sensed the energy shift just before, and again I did nothing, like all those other moments I sensed the energy shift with Dad.

A few years later after we moved out of the city. We moved for numerous mental health reasons: My dog because he had a biting-people problem. My husband because he had no-boundaries-with-work and drug problems. Dad, who had recently come into my life again and I wanted to see more of, but he had the city-makes-him-crazy problem. Then there was me who just wasn't happy because I had a take-on-other-people's-feelings problem.

It was our first Christmas in our new dream home. I was excited to have everyone I loved together in my home: my husband, Mom, my younger half-sister, and Dad.

Although tension was high between John and me, I made sure everyone was happy and taken care of on that Christmas day. The tree was perfectly decorated, the presents were wrapped, the food was prepared, and *The Nutcracker* played in the background as a reminder of my youthful days of dreaming and dancing as a Sugar Plum Fairy.

After Dad left, we all got in our pj's and cuddled on the couches to watch the movie *Inception*. Mom was moving around a lot and being a bit animated. John went upstairs and seemed somewhat irritated by being around everyone, and the dog was sleeping on the floor next to Mom's feet. Mom seemed restless and wanted the dog up with her. She wanted to wake him up to get him up on the couch with her, so she decided to do this by putting her face in his face. Bad idea. In a split second, he lunged at her and grabbed her lip. She was stunned and didn't quite know what happened. She ran to the bathroom. I scolded Newks; he knew immediately he did a bad, bad thing. Then I followed her. She was bleeding badly, and her lip did not look good. I panicked. My sister was stunned too. I knew Mom had to go to the hospital to get stitches, but I needed help making that call. I went to wake up John and somehow the plan quickly became that everyone got in the car to go to the hospital. I was left home alone with the pup while *Inception* still played in the background. I somehow felt stuck in my own nightmare of past experiences of sensing these energy shifts, my curse if you will.

What do these all have to do with Fear? Good question.

I have been curious about this thread that connects these stories since my healing session last year when all these memories linked together with my mom's Fear and my dad's Anger.

In all the scenarios, I was safe, but there was someone else that was not, and I always sensed it. Another thread is that I sensed it every time, except this last one with Mom. I believe this was because I was in a state of denial about many aspects of my life at that time and wasn't seeing the agitation that was all around me in my marriage.

This is where Fear lies. Fear of my knowing, Fear of my curse being that I could sense the energy shifts and not control them, or worse, that I was the one making them happen. All those moments, including the moments with Dad when he went on the attack, I thought about how agitated I was, how I felt the tension in my body, and how I sensed the change in the air seconds before it told me to take cover or someone else was about to go down.

I had other times where I sensed bad things were going to happen, so often that I started to speak up, or rather freak out. It usually came with lots of tears and me begging the person not to get in the car or make plans to go somewhere or to leave suddenly. If the person or people didn't listen, I would create such a scene with uncontrollable tears and the shaking of my body as I grasped on to hold them as if it might be the last time they left my side. Even in the moments all parties involved (including myself) thought I was crazy, somehow, I believed my wild pre-actions diverted the dark moment that was to come and moved it along to somewhere else. That was my tactic for a little while. Then, when my sanity was in question, I went back to just looking away.

So, Fear was closely linked with my intuition. The two in a twisted dance with each other. The cycle was this: I felt bad things were about to happen, then they did, and I began to fear I knew when other things might happen too. Whether I believed I was creating them or just tapped into something that was warning me didn't matter; it was all a curse and a reason to be afraid.

However, over time, I began to realize I was also tapped into the good stuff too. I would sense when my number would be called for a callback in a room full of 200 other dancers. I would walk in and just know when it was my day. I sensed good news was coming the day of my marriage proposal even though we spoke of not getting married. I sensed I would be offered a job in a matter of months, that our offer would be accepted on our dream house, and so many other beautiful moments of my life that I was tapped into. As I write this, I feel in my bones that this is going to touch you. In a way, it is reaching to a place you have also hidden deep within, maybe even from yourself, and I am inviting you to bring it out in the open to explore it now.

It wasn't until just recently I realized my intuition is and always has been a gift, not a curse. There were times I was tuned in but ignored it because I was afraid of what bad might come, or because I still wanted to have an element of awe and surprise when the good things happened. What was the most challenging was to discern when it was intuition and when it was Fear after the trauma I endured. My past haunted me, and I was just waiting for another metaphorical dog bite or the other shoe to drop. Fear was always on the lookout for these possible scenarios. I didn't trust myself, and if I didn't trust myself, how could I trust anyone else?

Aside from my fear of sensing those bad things on the horizon, the root fear for me has always been abandonment: not feeling seen, heard, felt, or taken care of by others. As I write this my whole body is so tense with the thought that this might get published *(spoiler alert, if you are reading this, it did!),* or no one reads it *(again, at least one person is, it's you! Thank you!),* and maybe worse, the person reading it doesn't care or doesn't resonate with it *(I hope it does because you somehow made it this far! But if it doesn't, I will still survive.)*

What Are We Afraid of?

Fear is based on evidence from the past and anticipating a possible negative outcome in the future.

In the philosophy of yoga, we tend to have conversations around the idea that all fear is based in the root fear of death. So, if you are afraid of something, it usually can be traced all the way to the possibility of death. One of my teachers uses the example of the fear of public speaking. What could go wrong? Well, aside from possibly walking out to the podium, falling off the stage, breaking your neck, and dying, the mind could always unconsciously trace the path to dying. The speech flops, you don't get any more speaking engagements, the company who you were representing lays you off because it was so bad. So, you lose your home, and you become an embarrassment to your family and friends. You become homeless from that awful speech you gave, and you fall asleep in the streets in the cold winter and die of hypothermia. You are dead so don't even bother with that speech; you know how it's going to end anyway.

We have a lot less to be afraid of in our cushy Western modern world, but our mind still looks out for the danger, especially if we are a person who never had a safe environment as a child and/or a survivor of trauma. We become hypervigilant for the sake of our survival.

When we speak about fear, we touch on the autonomic nervous system, which is composed of the sympathetic nervous system (what we call fight-flight-freeze-fawn) and the parasympathetic nervous system (what we call rest and digest). When we are in a heightened state of stress or fear, this triggers our fight or flight response. Our body releases stress hormones like adrenaline and cortisol and temporarily shuts down other systems like digestion and reproduction to focus on the task at hand in a state of stress. We need this if our body is in great danger. However, in our world today, we are constantly in a state of activating the sympathetic nervous system by stress and fear, and it is important to regulate and restore the body so that it can function more efficiently without going into fight or flight. If it does not, there can be long-lasting effects like digestive or reproductive problems because the body has shut them down to a certain extent.

When you are feeling scared, it is important to first acknowledge whether you are in fact safe in your body and your environment. When that is confirmed, take a moment to pause and listen to your body. If the heart is beating fast and breath is fast and shallow, it is important to slow down the breath to slow the heart rate and rest in a position that feels safe and supported. Ask yourself how you would prefer to feel in your physical body and in your emotional and thinking bodies. Is there something that could help you shift that? Maybe listen to a calming song to slow down the breath, so you can listen to what your body needs at that moment.

Simply ask, "What do I need?" This answer should be one to three words at most if it's coming from a place in your body. If it is rambling on, that is the mind chatter and ego. Take a few more slow breaths and listen again. By doing this, the body shifts into the relaxation response which is documented to change the physiology of the body. When the relaxation response switch is flipped, it turns on the parasympathetic nervous system, rest and digest. Practices like restorative yoga, yin yoga, meditation, and other passive practices intrinsically activate this relaxation response. This is particularly important in the modern world when we are under constant stress by our man-made expectations to live up to societal standards. The fight or flight response is always working at least at a steady hum which leads to the chronic diseases which we see increasing every day.

At The Root of Fear

Something I heard in a yoga class really shifted my perspective about the root of fear. As my teacher was speaking about fear and setting us up in a pose to feel physically grounded and safe and allow ourselves to move the energy of fear through our bodies, a man in class chimed in and offered us this: He explained that there is a Japanese character for Fear which translates to "mis-aligned." As I try to fact-check with my Google search skills, I do not find confirmation of this. However, I feel that back then it deeply resonated with me. I feel there is truth to what he shared, and it feels necessary to include it here for you to sit with.

Just think of it for a moment, when you were last afraid of something, was it because you did not quite feel aligned with it? Maybe it was because you were thinking something bad or unsafe could happen, and your natural state did not want to be aligned with it. Or maybe it was something you really wanted but were afraid about putting yourself out there and failing or maybe even succeeding. Still, your natural state was not feeling aligned with it yet.

In terms of the subtle energy body, the chakra system, we have the root chakra, which is at the root of our spine and pelvis and includes our legs and feet. Fear needs to be expressed here when we must get up and run or fight back if our life is at stake, but even more so back in our caveman days when we had to fight for our dinner or fight for our lives, so we were not dinner.

Energetically, this is where we not only feel safe, but also experience stability, or lack thereof if it is out of balance. We might not literally need to fight for our life, but we might not feel safe in other ways, like in sharing our words with someone, how we feel receiving someone else's harmful words, how our necessities are not being met like food or a safe home, or how we feel when we are not being supported by our loved ones. These scenarios can keep us in this state of fear until our basic need to feel safe again is met. This is important to recognize because we have a society built to keep us in a state of fear through news, religion, and politics whether you are conscious of it or not. Just think about how your nervous system feels after you watch the news or scroll through social media.

Why I emphasize the abandonment piece so much is that it was part of my story and I think it is a huge part of many people's stories about fear and not feeling safe. If our basic needs are not met and we feel abandoned by our parents, employers, community, or government, then we will remain in an unbalanced state at the root chakra and a heightened state in the sympathetic nervous system. Once you feel you can support and provide a safe space for yourself both in your body and your home, the root chakra and the nervous system can come back into balance.

Let's Check In

What are you afraid of? Does Abandonment also haunt you in the shadows?

Take a few minutes to sit with Fear in meditation. Try to visualize something that you are mildly afraid of but will not trigger you into a full-blown fearful and anxious state so you can really be the observer.

Observe:

- What does it feel like in your body?
- Are there certain places it sits in your body?
- Are there certain situations, archetypes of people, places, that it hangs out with?

Take three grounding breaths to release anything that may have come up and acknowledge yourself in the present moment where you are safe.

Repeat the mantra, "I am safe" for as long as you need, using your breath, to feel rooted again. You can do this any way that feels good for your body to receive the mantra. I often breathe in "I am" and exhale "safe" but you can also say the entire mantra on the inhale and again on the exhale.

Then get a pen and paper/journal.

- Begin to write a letter to Fear as I did at the beginning of this section. Address anything from your meditation that feels like it is an obstacle.

Now, here is a really cool part of the exercise that I have to give a big shout-out to Elizabeth Gilbert for. I had the privilege of seeing her and Rob Bell talk a few days after the 2016 election where the first half of the day was hijacked by the election results and how we would move forward as a nation. It was powerful and I often look back at my notes from that day.

One of the exercises we did in that workshop was to write a letter to Fear. Writing letters never sent to people, situations, or feelings was something I did quite often in my development. But this next step was a huge game-changer, at least with Fear (and feel free to repeat this with any of our other emotions throughout this book).

- Write your letter TO Fear then,

- Write a letter FROM Fear. Hear what it has to say through your pen. Don't get in the way, let it flow...

- Take a few breaths and reflect for a moment.

- Ask yourself, *whose voice was that?* Listen and see who comes through.

- Then, write one more letter back to Fear for resolution.

Now, here are a few healthy resources you can practice and use when you feel Fear's voice in your ear.

Centering Practices. These are for when you feel Fear is taking you off your center and about to spiral you into disorientation.

- This can be done wherever you want to feel safe in your body again. Place your hands on your body (heart, legs, whatever needs anchoring). Take five to ten long, easy breaths.

- Say the mantra "I am safe" as you take your breaths. Keep going if you still don't feel safe. The mantra can be said out loud or in your head and can be done with or without your hands on the body.

Containment Practices. If you still need a bit of help grounding your body so Fear doesn't trigger the stress hormones to fight or flight, try one of these.

- Use your hands to squeeze legs, feet, arms, shoulders—wherever you feel the stress of Fear taking over— to feel safe.

- Tighten and relax the muscles of your body (scan body from feet to head). This can be done lying down, if possible, seated or standing.

Now, whatever you are feeling in this moment, finish this statement:

As I release Fear and Abandonment, my body tells the story of...

Letter to Anger and Resentment

Dear Anger and Resentment,

Anger, I was never safe to feel you. I watched my dad get injected by you, and he hurt people. He turned into a monster within seconds when he was no longer in control of you. I felt you in me a few times as a child and it scared me too. I ended up feeling ashamed of myself because of the things I felt and did from your uncontrollable wrath. I threw innocent pets and stuffed animals into the walls simply because I did not know how to express you as a child by witnessing my dad. I always regretted my actions and cried tears of Shame and Guilt. As an adult, I didn't like being around you or having you in me, so I avoided being around you as much as I could and when you showed up, I buried you deep inside where you became the silent killer: Resentment.

Resentment, you lurked in the shadows of my marriage. I avoided Anger so much that I attracted someone who didn't know how to express his Anger either, which made him carry his own heavy load of Resentment. I felt you unconsciously in our daily conversations and as I look back, I can see how much he loathed me, and perhaps I loathed him too in moments when I didn't feel seen by him. We resented each other for not being what we wanted the other to be, or rather not be, which held us both back from being our authentic selves, at least for me. I felt a tremendous amount of you these past eight years after doing so much inner work and still not feeling seen or heard. You have now become my greatest obstacle from connecting with my Self, creating for the joy of it, and trusting others in authentic connections.

I resent YOU, Anger and Resentment! What the hell do you want from me?? Do you want me to experience your red-hot heat? For what? Do you want to keep me in your burning red flames? I don't want that for myself, and I am better than you both. There is way more to me than your one dimension. Anger, you are reactionary and mindless. You are a low-ball emotion. Resentment, you are a silent killer. My body does not deserve to house you after all the beautiful work she has done in this lifetime to create a sacred home for me.

You both caused pain in my body with urinary tract infections, fibroids, and acne. I take responsibility for not looking at you when you showed up in my body as a sign to look closer at my life, but I do not want you or need you here anymore. We need to find common ground.

Anger, if you come, I will honor you on my own terms, not with mindless hurtful words or actions towards myself or others. I will express you safely through movement, dance, and written words where it is safe to be released. I will not harbor you only to transform you into Resentment in my body again.

Resentment, you are never welcome here again. I will not blame others for what I feel I lack. I am special. What I do here is creative and I will not allow you to get in my way ever again by making me feel like I am not good enough. I will not resent people who seemingly burned me in my past, or anyone who is here now or who comes into my life to show me something that I still need to look at within myself. You have blocked people from loving me with your friend Fear for way too long.

You don't get to stay in this journal where I share my dreams. Thank you both for your time and what you taught me; I do not want your services anymore.

With deep gratitude,

Phoebe

Tears Flow to Block the Anger

For so many years, I thought I did it. I thought I was the one who created those angry moments with Dad. I carried the weight of him almost pulling the trigger on Mom, the beating of his girlfriend Katie, the moments when I felt like I "asked for it" when I was thrown into the sticks and the walls. I wished him away so many times because I was angry at him for messing up my life and then one day, he was gone. I thought all of this came true *because* of my anger. I was angry at the people in my life and angry at myself because I was too scared to speak up, but I still somehow had the power to manifest the emotive scenarios I was experiencing in the world.

This feeling of anger was a curse and I had to bury it deeply. I attracted men who didn't know how to express it either, where it was safer to have them just leave. Fights with boyfriends and my husband usually started with heated words and the moment the tone and volume escalated, the tears came from me, and they fled. They left me in my home, they left me at parties, they left me on the streets of New York City in the middle of one of the coldest nights of the year to walk home alone thirty blocks, and they left me at the lowest moment of my life, while grieving for the death of my dad. It was all a reflection of how I didn't know how to express Anger and it always seemed better to walk away from the tensions, so that I didn't create another scenario like the ones from childhood, or worse.

So, I buried these feelings of Anger, but the tears always came up to the surface, like a hydrothermal explosion. The healthiest way I knew to release Anger consciously was through sadness. It sometimes helped. But throughout my divorce, the tears were not doing the trick and my body was too emotionally exhausted. As I began to unpack my marriage and why he left me when he did, I became aware of Resentment that had been lurking in the shadows and it grew, it grew in my body to a breaking point which was the first time I felt like my body was going to give out.

Pissed Off

In August, seven months after Dad died, five months after John said he wanted a divorce, we signed our divorce papers. We had nothing to bind us except our dog. The night we signed the papers, we went out for a drink to "celebrate." The bartender probably thought we were completely mad when we told her what we were celebrating, and it was probably the most fun we had together in a few years. We laughed about the insanity of our lives without the pressure of being attached to any expectations of each other anymore. We were both pretty intoxicated. When he walked me to my place, he got serious and he said that I could keep my dad's estate money, that I didn't owe him anything when it came through, *(Wait, what? No shit buddy!)* and within the same breath, he said he was making a conscious choice to not change. He decided to continue the path of self-destruction and anyone who comes along was going to go down with him. He got in his car intoxicated and drove home. I felt my heart breaking for him as he drove off but was also pissed that I had to still carry the weight of this secret of his. I knew I was going to be the one who would still know that the girl he was seeing would be as ignorant as I was—maybe more so because I knew about the drug use but chose to look away—and now, I couldn't do anything.

The man that I was seeing that summer, The Chef, came over after work. He was also a bit tipsy. We probably also shared a drink or two. My dog, Newkie, was annoyed at us both for being kind of loud and giddy. The Chef did the worst thing that he could have probably done, especially now that you know about Newks. He put his face in the dog's face while Newkie was lying down, and just like that, Newkie went in for the lip, again. It all happened so fast, yet *again* I knew it was going to happen. I felt the uneasy tension from the night in my body, which the dog always picked up on, and I chose to ignore it, again. The Chef immediately popped up and grabbed his lip, to see if it was there. Most of it was, but there was a very small piece on my bedroom floor, next to the bedside table. I threw my dog across the room and tended to The Chef. I got a towel to put pressure on to stop the bleeding. I yelled at my dog, and he shied into a corner with his tail curled up between his legs. He knew and was already ashamed. The incident sobered me up and I drove us to the hospital, the same one Mom went to just nine months prior. We ended up being there for a few hours while he got stitches over his lip.

I called John the next day to let him know what was going on. He said we had to put the dog down. I cried for my pup. As much as I tried to find an alternative the following weeks, I eventually went along with his decision. I wasn't in a living situation where I could have him run around free or monitor my guests, and John had no desire to keep him in his life. He arranged with our vet to put him down in two weeks. It would be another door closing on any connection with John.

The next weekend, I had booked a retreat for myself. It was during the time away that I began to realize how I wasn't taking care of myself as much as I had been before and that I had put my needs aside for others, yet again. There was a fine balance of the energies those years after my dad entered back into my life. I felt drained by the past trauma of being around my dad, fearing he would snap if he was triggered. There was the constant pleasing of John, trying to make enough money so he thought I was worthy in his eyes, and making sure he was also in a good mental state so he would not use again. All of this unconsciously outweighed the love I had for both of them. Their love should have filled me up again, but it didn't. Then after all the loss, I was empty. That weekend, I took myself out for a fancy dinner, got a massage and a facial (my skin was getting bad with severe breakouts), and I took a long, sensual bath in the clawfoot bathtub of the bed and breakfast. It was healing but also made me mad at how much I neglected myself. I felt resentful for the lost time with myself.

The following weekend was Labor Day weekend. The Chef came to spend the night. We both knew it was ending since he was moving back to Brooklyn at the end of the month. His lip was still red from the stitches where my dog had bitten him a couple of weeks prior. We had sex for the last time and took a shower together the next morning before he left. As he cleaned himself off, he remarked that something felt off in my body and warned me to pay attention. The next day I woke up in terrible pain because I had a UTI. It was Monday, Labor Day, and all the doctors ' offices were closed, even urgent care. I was working at the hotel front desk most of the day and writhed in pain. By the time my shift was over around 4:00 p.m., I drove myself to the ER after Mom texted to urge me to go before it turned into a kidney infection.

I drove myself back to the same hospital I had just taken The Chef to and now I was the patient. I was in severe pain, and they asked if I wanted morphine. I declined, knowing I would have to drive myself home once they figured out what was wrong. They were concerned that my pain was more than a UTI, so they ran a few tests and confirmed I also had a kidney stone in my right kidney. After a few hours there, they gave me an antibiotic for the UTI and sent me home. The pain subsided a little and I got a bit better the rest of the week. I continued back to work as normal and made plans for Mom to come to visit me on Sunday to help me put down my dog since John insisted that even though he was the one who wanted to have him put down, he was too busy to go with me.

The Saturday night before, I had Newkie with me. I was supposed to go out to meet The Chef at his last event, but I canceled. I still wasn't feeling great. I fell asleep at 8:00 p.m. and woke up screaming in pain a little before midnight.

The waves of pain streamed through me every fifteen minutes, like I was about to either give birth or die. It was a piercing pain in my abdomen. It was as if there was something inside of me that had massive claws and was dying to come out and rear its ugly head. I was sweating profusely and was shivering at the same time. I didn't know what to do but knew I should probably get myself to the toilet to let whatever was inside of me out. It took what felt like hours to crawl to the bathroom each time the waves of pain came, and I peed blood. *It isn't my period. What is it? It cannot be the UTI; I am on antibiotics.*

My pup paced back and forth and looked at me with such concern. He wanted to do something for me, but he didn't know what. If he were bigger, I imagine he would have tried to carry me, but the thirty-pound scrawny-legged guy wasn't able to. Each time I screamed as I gave birth to pee that felt like shards of glass, Newkie put his head on my lap and looked up at me with the saddest, most helpless eyes. He felt my pain and wanted to help me, his owner, his love, the human he trusted most. Little did he know that same person would be taking his life in just a matter of days. At that moment, I wasn't sure which outweighed the other: my guilt, my anger toward John for making me put this lovable creature down, or my physical pain.

The waves of pain lasted until late morning and then I just felt like general crap the rest of the day. I texted John to see if he could help take care of Newks since I was clearly in no shape to walk him down the stairs of my apartment building and outside when I could barely crawl to my bathroom, but he was away for the weekend with his girlfriend. I managed to get clothes on and walk Newks to the end of my street. He was on his best behavior, took care of business immediately, and did not make any contact with a potential victim.

As I came out of the waves of pain and consulted with friends who had passed kidney stones before, I concluded I passed the kidney stone doctors saw just days before.

Mom arrived later that afternoon to help prepare our last days with Newkie and thankfully, was also able to aid me back to health. I started to feel much better. Monday, I thought it would be nice to get my name changed back to Miller, my maiden name, to rid me of my married past and honor my deceased Dad. It felt good to start with a clean slate. After I taught in the morning, Mom and I headed up to Poughkeepsie to yet another courthouse. I knew them well by this time that year, between my divorce and dealing with my dad's estate.

I was done with my married name, I wanted nothing more to do with it. The next day would be the last of my connections to John, his name as my own and our dog would be put to rest. While I was at work the following day,

Mom took Newks to the vet and held him until his very last breath. It was best that I wasn't there. She told him how loved he was and made sure he was able to fall asleep peacefully. She was happy she could be there for him to transition to another life.

We had a little ceremony with a couple of my friends that evening. The next day, I got up to get ready to work as Mom prepared for her drive back home. Moments before I was supposed to leave, the wave of pain started again and this time it felt even worse. I fell to the floor in the fetal position and screamed, "It's happening again!!" Mom insisted we go to the ER, but I couldn't move and didn't want to move. I probably thought it would be best to just die right there and then. I somehow managed to cancel my class and got in the car. Mom drove me to the ER as I battled with crying and holding it back because it only made the pain worse. They admitted me right away and immediately gave me morphine. It was the first time I ever had an IV, and I thought that I was peeing myself as I felt the fluids travel throughout my body. Then it was a beautiful feeling of warmth where everything was soft and easy. It was like nothing I had experienced before. I was beginning to understand why people liked drugs so much. The pain just went away.

We were there for hours as they ran various tests that poked and prodded my body. One doctor looked at my chart and said I still had the kidney stone that I thought I had passed, another said it was probably ovarian cysts, another wanted to rule out appendicitis, and another had no idea what was going on inside of me. Once I was stabilized, they finally sent me home with referrals to my gynecologist and a urologist. I would spend the next two months in and out of doctors' offices trying to figure out what happened. For about a month I had the waves of pain at the same time every morning at the same place, my lower right abdomen. I reached out to my acupuncturist who shared that it was the time of day when the body was cleansing the heart. I was trying to clear my heart of the pain.

Around this same time, my skin was getting bad, cystic acne that was painful, and it was hard to look at myself. I remember going into the bathroom at work and not being able to look in the mirror. If I did happen to catch my eye, I winced in pain. I occasionally return to that public restroom at my old job, remembering those days, and tell myself, "We have come a long way, Phoebe."

Every morning for the next month or so, I had a hard time recognizing myself in my bathroom mirror. Although I saw the same sad reflection in the mirror, I no longer knew who I was looking at. I felt like I wanted to peel off my skin and scream. I wanted to run away. I was deeply sad, hurt, and what I didn't realize, *very angry*. Every week my therapist asked me if I was angry. I didn't feel I had the energy to be angry, and I didn't even know at that point whom to be angry at.

I also wasn't sure how I was going to keep moving forward with my job. It was my only stability, my anchor, but it was becoming more and more of a heavy weight that seemed to be pulling me down. The place was toxic. People gossiped and complained about everything. While I was trying to do my best to keep my head above water, I was feeling the pressure to drown in their toxicity. I wasn't sure how to get free from that obstacle.

When Mom was visiting around the time of her birthday, my boss insisted I come in for an all-company meeting on my one night off. I was peeved since it was Mom's birthday and we had to rearrange our plans. The meeting had nothing to do with my department, but I still went. My boss acknowledged all the members of management but forgot to include me, the director of the yoga program. Apparently, the only reason I was supposed to be there was to represent my department so she could introduce me. Her father whispered to her later and she laughed off an apology to me. It was clear to me how she felt about me and my department: not worth mentioning or worth her time.

A few days later I had to go to yet another follow-up exam for my mysterious episodes of pain. I had to leave work early, but before I left, I was determined to have a meeting with my boss. I was always last on her list if I was on it at all. On my way out, she said she was disappointed in my performance and that I was "just not the same anymore." I was so heated by her comment because of course, I wasn't the same. I was also upset that I would never be able to be the same ever again after the year that had stripped everything from me, including who I knew myself to be. I was angry at the entire Universe for giving me such a crap sandwich of life.

I went to get physically poked at again after my boss poked at my emotional wellbeing. I sat with my feet in stirrups with, yet another camera crammed up inside of me. The woman who was monitoring it was very talkative. She asked if I planned to have kids. I had not thought about it being newly single and having no prospects in front of me. Kids were the least of my thoughts then. She said, "Well if you do, you might want to get it all checked out because I see a potential problem," but she was not at liberty to tell me anything. Still in a bad mood from my boss, I was horrified by the news. Even if I wasn't sure, how dare she try to scare me out of having children. It was yet another thing to add to the list of things I could potentially lose.

That night I had dreams laced with so much anger. I was going back and forth between being tortured by John and my boss. I was doing my best to retaliate. When I woke up, I had immediate dread. I didn't want to move. I didn't want to go back to that toxic place and feel ignored again. My little studio was my haven where students were loving and supportive but just outside the elevator doors was a swamp of despair.

I texted Mom, "Can I come home this weekend?"

Within seconds, "YES!"

A minute went by, I wrote, "Can I come home tomorrow?"

She immediately replied, "Sure! Even better."

I took a breath, "Can I come home now?"

She didn't even take a beat, "Come home, Phoebe."

During the drive to Mom's, I decided to leave my job. The next week when I returned, I gave my notice and within a month or so, I found myself living in Costa Rica for nine months to begin my recovery.

It took me a few years to really face my anger which eventually manifested into resentment where it settled into my body, again. It took another wave of heartbreaks to get it, before I found a healthy way to give it expression.

I attracted two passionate relationships where I fell in love and at the expense of them, I allowed myself to feel angry. I took a lot of my past out on these two men who my girlfriends respectfully named Peter Pan and San Diego. Any little moment that triggered my abandonment wound turned into full-blown disasters between Peter Pan and me.

When San Diego came around, I resisted at first since we were dear friends, then I fell in love, hard. I was scared of feeling so strongly for someone who could potentially hurt me, so I pushed him away. He went away a few times, but he always came back. It was like I needed him to pass some kind of test to win my heart, a test I had never given to anyone else before. I tested him as if he was all those men before him all over again. I called him out on his shortcomings and demanded he make changes, and he pretty much came through every time, although quite delayed which was a huge trigger for me, and I lashed out like an angry cat. I sometimes wondered if he was attracted to my angry streak, which didn't feel like me. By then I lived by the rule, "You can't say the wrong thing to the right person." And I tested it with him. I said everything I wanted to say to all the wrong people before him and figured if he stayed, then he was the right guy for me.

The breaking point was when I demanded he get a divorce from his ex, with whom he was amicably separated and co-parenting. I wanted to know there was space for me and the possibility for us to have a family. He dragged his feet too long and the red alarms went off, "abandon ship!!!" I was triggered. I gave him a timeframe to take steps towards a divorce to show me he was making an effort and he didn't do it. I no longer felt safe in trusting him, and I had to build trust in myself by staying true to my word. We broke up. I closed the door on the relationship with a lot of pain and anger in my heart.

A few months went by, he came back. San Diego told me he made moves towards his divorce to be with me again. I didn't trust him, and I was still hurt from all the rejection from the past several years by men. It was too much, and I left San Diego in his mom's car in the parking lot, the same lot where we made plans to have our first date a couple of years earlier.

Within days, I had another UTI. I dealt with them on and off the rest of that winter into spring. I felt confused and missed San Diego again. I reached out to him to see if we could work something out. He had the upper hand now. He had moved on, was now dating someone, and wanted nothing to do with me.

Rejection again filled me with rage. My body felt all the years I had been rejected, the back and forth, the highs and lows, it all came to a head. I wanted to get it out but didn't know the first thing to do with it. In that same parking lot, where I left San Diego six months earlier, I called my healer as a follow-up to our first session where she talked me off a ledge. I felt like I wanted to strip my skin off my body and burn it to shreds. She said I needed to let it flow, not to fight it, and get angry, scream, attack a pillow, write a nasty letter, anything. I got off the phone and screamed until my face was burning red and my body shook to the core from the adrenaline. It was just the beginning of the release, but it was already deep inside me, brewing.

The UTIs were there for another year, no matter what I did. Antibiotics weren't doing anything, so I turned to alternative medicine which kept them from full raging. I also woke up one morning with a rash on my face that stayed there for a good year or so. Every morning, I felt the bumps on my face the moment I woke up, hoping that it was all just a bad dream. When I looked in the mirror, I confirmed it was still there, a bright red, flush, and irritation for everyone to see. I could not hide it with makeup. It was a constant reminder of what I was feeling inside. My periods were also getting worse, with so much cramping that I needed to take about four Advil every four hours on my second and third days of bleeding.

A Bloody Mess

After about a year of inner work, acupuncture to release the heat, other numerous healers of various modalities, and Western doctors, the symptoms slowly improved. I started to intentionally invite things that brought me joy into my life again, like dancing and writing. I even created a movement practice to heal and my podcast to share other people's stories. I began to feel a shift in my world and my body began to reflect it. Until…

A year later, I went to visit my gramma after her knee surgery. My half-sister Willa and I surprised her with a visit to take care of her one weekend since other family members were tied up. I got there and right away, I started to bleed.

We watched an episode of *Queer Eye for the Straight Guy* and the man they were making over reminded me for some reason of San Diego. He was a father, and you could tell he loved his daughter. It made me think about what we could have had together. We both joked that if we had a daughter together, he would be a lost cause and that he would be such a big pushover for her.

Feeling the heaviness in my heart, I got up, went to the guest bathroom, and immediately an intense wave of pain came on strong, fast, and intense. I started to cry and moan, I remember thinking, *if this is what giving birth feels like, I never want to have a baby.* I didn't know where exactly that thought came from, but the contraction-like waves of pain took me down to the ground and I stayed there for a little while. I managed to crawl to my room when my sister came in to check on me. I asked her to get a few Advil from

Gramma's bathroom, I took them and immediately fell asleep. The pain knocked me out cold. When I woke, I felt as if something had been lifted from my body. Maybe it was the Advil, maybe it was the waves that cracked me open for it to be removed. I was just grateful to be relieved of the burden I had felt.

My mom had arrived, and I went out to say hello. I looked down at my phone that had been out in the living room during my episode and saw a message from San Diego that had come in. It was an email that confirmed something, and I intuitively felt he had gotten the person he was seeing pregnant, and she was keeping it.

The episode I had just thirty minutes prior, was somehow a direct reflection of that email that I felt him typing on the other side of the country. There was no other way to explain it. I felt the waves of pain in my heart this time. That door would forever be closed on us. There was no going back, no possibility of having a family with him while he was going to have a new one of his own. I was angry at myself for being such a fool to have held onto that possibility for so long, almost two years from our initial break up. What was I thinking? Or better yet *why* was I allowing myself to obsessively think about him so much while I wasn't listening to my body? It was screaming out to me to let that pain go!

I continued to have these types of episodes during my period that somehow replicated the sensations of my mysterious UTI episodes six years prior. They escalated and were unpredictable (aside from them only showing up while I was menstruating). After one of them one morning, I had a doctor's appointment for something else. I had passed out on the bathroom floor after a few hours of feverishly vomiting in a trash bag while bleeding like a faucet and shitting on the toilet.

I somehow dragged myself to the doctor's appointment. I think it was the heated seats to comfort the cramps that convinced me I could make it. The nurse took one look at me and asked what was wrong. She felt my clammy hands and told me to make sure I let the doctor know, even if that wasn't the purpose of my visit. When he walked in, I told him I was super weak and tried to explain what happened. He looked at me with little pitiful eyes and said, "Oh, cramps? That's too bad" and went on to address the other issue I came in for. I wanted to reach out and grab him by his stethoscope, wrap it around his neck and say "No, you fucking idiot! I feel like I just gave birth to a devil child that clawed its way out of me for two hours" but because I felt so damn weak, I just said, "Yeah, cramps."

These episodes went on for months. After seeing my gynecologist, who was way more understanding than the idiot male doctor, she recommended I get a D&C after confirming that I had fibroids and an ovarian cyst. She also suspected endometriosis but could not confirm that. She requested to do it immediately, but I had plans to lead a retreat in Bali, so it got scheduled upon my return for April 6, 2020. That was before we knew that COVID would be a thing that would shut our world down as we knew it. The surgery was canceled indefinitely so I had to take matters into my own hands.

Cooling Off

I started an Ayurvedic cleanse and reached out to a few trusted healer friends who could offer their services online. It was three months of a grueling cleanse to take the heat out of my system that seemed to be the root cause of the menstruating episodes, the ongoing skin issues, and the low-grade UTIs. On the other side of it, I felt like I took a turn for the better. My symptoms significantly improved, mostly the skin and UTIs, and the episodes with my period were much smaller waves of pain.

During these months, I was living with my gramma after I chose to be closer to my family through the pandemic. It was nurturing, challenging, and overall, the best thing that could have happened for my healing. In fact, the pandemic for me was a blessing in many ways because it took so much of the external triggers away but also put me front and center with the roots of my pain. I had the chance to see the family dynamics in a new light.

I got closer with my gramma which gave me a new perspective but did not always bring out the best in me. She is a perfectionist and at times she put that on me. We got into an argument one day about something happening in the world of politics and how it was affecting our family, and I started screaming at her. I said, "Gramma, you expect too much from us! You do that because you do that to yourself. It hurts me to see that you don't see how beautiful you really are!" That moment, the energy shifted from tension to a big sigh. I started to cry, and we held an embrace for so long. As I wept, she said, "My love, you are way deeper than I will ever be. You feel so much." That moment, I saw how much I was like her and at the same time how very different we both are.

During this time, I befriended a few male friends and made stronger bonds with them to slowly build my trust in men again. I started to be more vulnerable with them and they reciprocated, saying I was a safe person to share with.

It made me happy to know I was feeling at home again and that others felt at home with me too with no expectations.

Everything was feeling a bit easier, puzzle pieces were somehow falling gently into place integrating both in my body and my life. After several healing sessions, my BodyTalk facilitator received a message that there was a scar. She dug around for more information, and we were both convinced it was related to my healing of the last year.

In December, I ended up getting the D&C and I am grateful I did. Everything in that experience of my menstruation has shifted. I even see it as a gift now how my body is shedding a monthly cycle of my life that I no longer need and ebbs and flows with the moon. It wasn't a magic wand; it took some time after the surgery for my body to adjust.

As I reflect upon this eight-year journey with Anger and Resentment, I feel there has been great healing in listening to them more deeply. I listen to understand but not to get rid of. That is where I hit a wall before. I thought if I listened and understood, then they would kindly exit the building. This is not true. As I write this, another book of mine has just been released, a multi-author book that shares a little glimpse of this journey I have been sharing with you. The week it came out, I felt extremely angry again. I don't know why exactly. I had moments where I screamed, "I hate you!" not even knowing who "you" was supposed to be. There is something about knowing people are reading my words that is triggering old wounds as I *feel* people read them. I can subtly feel the thoughts and energy. Perhaps I feel angry because here I am eight years later, and I still don't know what I am doing and don't have the things I want most in my life just yet. I still want to have a healthy romantic relationship with a partner. I want to feel successful in how I help people and not feel like what I went through was just the way of life, but it was somehow purposeful for others. I want a home that feels like I have roots and like I belong in this world. Maybe I will receive all of it someday. I don't know.

What I do know is I can't resist Anger when it comes, I just have to let it flow, or else it is going to find a way to scream at me again. When it comes to my door now, I scream, I cry out "What the hell do you want from me?" I trust that something else is on the other side of it though, just like all the other times Anger and I danced together. There was always a break into creation. When I went through my great year of loss, I created a new company out of what I wanted to see for our world. After my breakup with San Diego, I created a podcast to share people's stories and a movement practice that helped me, and others, heal. So, when it comes again, I will just allow it to take me where I am going and trust I will create magic from it again.

There is So Much More to Anger

This was the one topic I thought would be short and sweet but as I wrote this it looks to be the one subject on which I have the most to say. As I have been writing these stories, I have been reliving them in my body. I found my jaw being held with tension like I used to feel when I held back my words during my marriage. Every few lines, I stopped, checked in, and reminded myself to release the tension in my jaw and keep typing. Anger is held in so many places in our bodies. I have demonstrated it through my story in many ways. In Chinese medicine, another place Anger is harbored is the liver. Wherever you may hold it, start to become aware in those moments you feel triggered. For our purposes here,

I am going to mostly speak into Anger because I feel that if Anger is not processed, Resentment can be one of the results. It goes on to become the silent killer in all the ways that Anger does, but just not so obvious, like my story.

It shows up differently in everyone. For example, I buried Anger and Resentment in my body, but you may be a loose cannon and blow off your steam into your world with venomous words and/or actions that will still come back to your body in some way. Perhaps from your hurtful words or actions towards someone, you feel the repercussions of Shame or Guilt or still harbor the unprocessed Anger that transforms into the silent killer, Resentment. We can numb ourselves to any of this in many ways. I like to use the example of alcoholism and drug abuse which ultimately attack the liver, through its processing and elimination of toxicity. I'm going to go out on a limb and say that most people with these diseases are harboring unprocessed anger whether it is the life that was dealt by their parents, society, or themselves, which is also wrapped up with Shame and Guilt. They don't know how to feel, or like me, are afraid to feel these feelings, so they numb the pain of Anger and Resentment by putting on a fake happy face and cracking open another bottle of gin.

My alcoholic grandparents harbored anger towards each other (for reasons I do not know), they made sure they had their gin and tonics ready by 3:00 p.m. and kept their refills flowing as they said their passive-aggressive comments until they went to bed. I guess these hours got earlier as they got older since I saw my grandfather at Dad's 11:00 a.m. funeral and he was already wasted. As he sipped his morning G&T with a shaky hand, he actually said, "It's too bad Jay never got sober." I wanted to leap across the table to strangle that man but then I sat back, paused, and listened again. My grandpa's name was also Jay and I wondered if perhaps it was his way of saying it about himself. Maybe he was angry that he never did, and my dad did, which kept the walls up in some way from really connecting with his son, *who knows?* That is their story now to work out in the life beyond here.

My dad was no doubt angry at himself for what he had to do in Vietnam. He told me stories after he was sober about the orders he had as a helicopter pilot to do whatever he needed to do to make sure he wasn't shot down, even if it meant sacrificing his own men. I read the psych documents he kept about the people he killed, women and children included. As an officer, he had the liberty to leave his post and go get the "good drugs" to numb himself from the anger he had towards himself for following through with orders. When heroin wasn't cutting it anymore, he shot himself in the leg in an attempt to get out of his hell. That was a story my dad finally worked through the last fourteen years of his life so he could finally die in peace.

I watched John struggle with alcohol and pill addiction throughout our marriage and never knew what to make of what I first thought was just a young, wild musician who eventually turned into a sad, angry, resentful man. Why he went down this spiral with Anger and Resentment, I don't know. That is his story to unfold if he ever chooses to do so.

I felt called to share these examples to show you that perhaps our Anger calls the body to the bottle in some way to numb it. Ultimately unprocessed Anger and Resentment still attack the body, and often through the liver, which is the organ to detoxify our poisons and venom. I'm not saying this is always the case. For others who are pulled to the bottle, maybe it was a heartbreak, a great loss that they numb, and they end life with a broken heart, a heart attack. These are just ways to look at the messages of the body again through a new lens.

Find Your Sacral Flow

In terms of our chakra system, I am going to invite us into the sacral chakra for a couple of reasons. In my own studies, I found conflicting information about where Anger and Resentment like to hang out in the body. The solar plexus, which is in the center of our torso, is suggested because the element of the energy is fire. When we get angry, we become heated, it feels like a great boiling, so that makes sense. As mentioned before in Chinese medicine, the liver, as well as the stomach, are the organs that hold unprocessed anger, and the solar plexus is where these organs reside. When there is too much heat, maybe that is again from unprocessed anger, in either of these organs, our bodies go haywire, so this also makes sense.

However, I also feel Anger likes hanging out in the sacral chakra, which is just below the solar plexus, our lower abdomen. You saw that clearly in my story of UTIs in the bladder, and fibroids in the uterus. Now, after many healings with many different practitioners, we also concluded that the heat from the solar plexus was infiltrating the other chakras, which I am also very open to believing. For instance, my skin condition could have been a result of the excess heat in my stomach and came up through my face as acne or rashes. I think this is a possibility.

I am going to offer one more way of looking at it that just came to me this week about the relationship between the sacral chakra and anger. This chakra is all about creation and our unique expression of the Self. This is where we give birth (literally) to new things. It is where Chaos resides, being a great void, or gap for creation. As I have been processing this latest angry bout of mine, I spoke at a women's group I am a part of about my present state and how I normally end up crying and being sad. A few women responded by saying how anger is a higher energy frequency and this is a good thing! I went to bed immediately after the group and woke up in a feverish state, crying, writing in an angry journal entry saying again, "I fucking hate you!" I exhausted myself into sleep and then woke up feeling better.

I had let the energy roll through me that night, and you know what was on the other side? A new result. A new way of figuring out a problem I was dealing with, a new way of seeing my situation, a new possibility of feeling happy. I took a breath of gentle, nurturing air and then paused. I quickly remembered those other moments. I felt the rage and anger boil inside of me. On the other side of the release of anger, there was some new creation of mine. After that horrible year of grieving my dad and divorce, I created nOMad, my company. After my breakup with San Diego, I created my healing somatic/movement practice, Mvt109™, and the podcast, "The Space in Between." Now, amid this present situation, I am creating this—my first solo book. Some of us might need that fire to fuel our creativity. I never knew it for myself but now I see it and want to look back to trace all the other little meltdowns of my life to something new that was born from it. I can see a few of them right now.

All that to say, the sacral chakra is the element of water, going with the flow, surrendering to the divine. Maybe that does work for some people or at some points in our lives. But maybe for other people or at other times in our lives, we just need to light the fire under our asses and create something great. Anger can get us there if we know how to use it and express it productively and creatively.

Let's Check In

It's important to first know what your triggers are, or the things that get you out of balance. What situations or relationships get you fired up?

- Is it when someone rejects your idea? Cuts you off in traffic? When someone speaks harsh words about people they don't understand and judges them?

- Is it relationships with men? Women? Romantic relationships? Family? With friends that test your boundaries?

- Take a few minutes to write down the last few times you felt angry or resentful about something.

Do you know why you felt triggered?

- How did it represent a situation or relationship from your past?

- What else was going on in your life where you could not fully express yourself?

- In what ways did anger feel like the safer way to deal with it?

Where did you feel it in your body?

- Did your face flush?

- Did your skin boil?

- A burning inside your gut?

- Did your body fire up and get jittery with adrenaline?

If you can't remember, take a few minutes (if you feel safe to go back there) and sit with the situation again and observe how the body responds. Below is an exercise that I use extensively since it was passed on to me by my teachers while I was dealing with the sensations of pain in my period.

Here and Now, I am Feeling.... (An original interoceptive awareness practice created by Elizabeth Andes-Bell and Bruce Bell, shared here with permission.)

This practice involves a huge energy shift in awareness and allows the release of attachments to thoughts, feelings, and expectations. This can be practiced alone wherever you are. Make sure to try this first in a neutral state but you can later work up using it in a state of tension. It can be a very valuable tool to recognize and release feelings of anger, anxiety, and fear.

- First, start by witnessing any sensations in the body.

- Without labeling them or identifying them as painful or pleasurable, state what you feel. Stay away from thoughts or emotions. Stick to sensations of the body. Get very descriptive. Start by stating to yourself "**Here and Now I am feeling...**"

    - A tight sensation in my chest

    - A fluttering in my stomach

    - A sharp sensation in my head

- Once started, take a couple of breaths, and watch again.

- Notice any change that has occurred. Watch the smallest shift and acknowledge it, give it words. Do the sensations feel less intense, more intense, dissipated, localized?

- Repeat until the sensation releases or changes until you feel satisfied.

- This practice can also be shared with a partner as a

conscious communication exercise to assist in expressing frustration, anger, resentment, or other challenging emotions that get in the way of healthy communication.

Other resources that can be helpful when experiencing anger in the body:

Gong and Sound Healing Meditations. These helped divert my vibration to a more positive one when I was feeling an episode come on. I think it can be helpful if you are in an intense state of any kind of unwanted vibration like pain or anger, to reset your vibration to a higher frequency to bring you back to homeostasis. There is so much research now about how sound healing and how listening to sounds at certain frequencies can heal the body.

Counting Breaths. When my dad came back into my life, although he was rehabilitated, he still got triggered. There was one day on my birthday we had an errand to run to get something for his phone. The salesperson was not understanding him, and Dad felt threatened; he started to tell himself a story that the guy had it out for him. Old feelings of wanting to take cover came to my body and I felt an "Uh-oh. We might get kicked out of here soon." I immediately had that familiar feeling of being paralyzed. But instead of his old ways of threatening to beat this guy's ass, I saw him starting to count on his hands and he was breathing. Within two breaths, he was calm and explained himself in a tone where nobody felt threatened, and we left with the device he needed. If you are one to get thrown into a loop of anger like my dad, slowly count your breaths and see how your body responds and let your mind catch up. You might find that it is not worth the energy to entertain anger at that moment. Also to note, when our emotions are triggered, it takes ninety seconds to move through the body, after that the mind takes over and continues to fuel the fire. If you can breathe it out for ninety seconds, watch what happens.

Dance, Sing, Scream it out. My absolute favorite. Give your anger expression. This is good if you are like me and don't know how to tap into anger for fear of what you might find there when you do. Put on a loud song and dance and scream, shout out what you don't feel safe saying to someone else, and let that shit go!

Write it out. The letter at the beginning of this section was a letter I wrote to release my dysfunctional relationship with Anger and Resentment. After I typed it here for you to see, I burned it to let it go. You can do this with a writing ritual for any emotion, to anyone with whom you have a complicated relationship. No need to send it to them; it's out there for you to release and no longer harbor it inside anymore. The most important thing is to **not** filter yourself and be clear with what you need to say. Then, if you feel called, burn it!!! Send it to the Universe to recycle into new energy.

Now, whatever you are feeling in this moment, finish this statement:

As I release Anger and Resentment, my body tells the story of...

Letter to Shame and Guilt

Dear Shame and Guilt,

So many men walked through my life that made me feel you both, which deeply hurt. There were multiple wounds and multiple ways I got to experience each of you. Mainly, I did things to push the men in my life away for fear of them seeing me. That hurt them, and I was left feeling guilty. Then as a repercussion, I would self-sabotage in other ways, and I was left feeling ashamed of myself. It was a vicious cycle, and it all began with Dad.

On that rainy night of my freshman year when I just could not take it anymore, I walked away; I couldn't be his lifeline anymore. I believed wholeheartedly then that if anything happened to him after that night, it would be on me, it would be my fault. Guilt, you held your grip on me for eighteen years. A fifteen-year-old somehow carried the weight and responsibility of all the years of her dad's suffering. I believed that absurd idea and you let me do it so you could have control over me. I now know that I wasn't responsible. I know that now. I am lucky that there was a positive outcome with Dad that freed me from you Guilt, otherwise, you may have eaten me alive.

There has been some weight of Guilt about abandoning my ex-husband with his disease even though he was the one who abandoned me and our marriage.

Consciously, I do know that he made his own choices to continue down a path of self-destruction. He is repeating patterns with someone else, giving himself the illusion that he is starting over with a clean slate. I know he chose to free us for both of our sakes in his way. I would like to think I did my best as a partner and wife but there is still a gnawing feeling sometimes that I failed him somehow. I am haunted in my dreams. This is where you lurked in the shadows deep within me, Guilt.

Shame, you have had such a way with me too. You came to me through Guilt and self-sabotage. I got to feel your painful sensations and humiliation at my core, repeatedly. I secretly wanted to suffer. I played the victim to feel your pain over and over again. I put myself in situations that were doomed from the start and would be "surprised" when my heart got broken. I secretly wanted to beg and plead, and would often cry out, "But I am a good person!" only to have you, Shame, make me feel like the unworthy person that I felt I should be. I was so unconscious of this cycle, but I watched it take its course and go rogue every time and would cry out, "Why am I here again?" I was convinced the last time I started to play this game that I was doing everything right, but I still ended up in the same place with you, Shame.

It wasn't until I looked back at the night when a stranger came inside of me that I realized it was time to release this story and break free from you both, Shame and Guilt. I allowed myself to be in that situation again and again, metaphorically, to feel that shame in various ways with the men in my life.

It wasn't until I really hurt someone I loved deeply and finally believed that someone loved me too, that I fully realized this. Because of that hurt I put upon us, he shut me out of his life and denied me his love for the last time. I knew I had to change. I knew I had to break this cycle with you. I knew if there was any sense of hope for me, I would have to forgive myself for leaving my dad, my ex, and for pushing away all the other men who came into my life to show me what love was. I had to learn how to love myself. That was the key to letting that tight fist in my abdomen loosen its grip. I didn't know how tight it was until it let go of me.

It was only a few months ago that I felt that gentle, yet quite deeply profound, release. Let me tell you Guilt and Shame, you are now a distant memory. I no longer feel your intense pangs of pain deep within me. Instead, I feel at ease and know in my bones that I am a good person who is worthy of love, both to give it and receive it. I feel free to love unconditionally without either of you haunting me anymore. You taught me valuable lessons. Your scars run deep but they are only little marks now of distant memories that I never need to cut open again.

With love and grace,
I release you both.

Phoebe

Guilty Non-Pleasures

I was mad at him. We were caught in a relationship cycle. It was a cycle I knew all too well already by the age of nineteen. It was the cycle of not feeling seen or heard but I kept being there for my emotionally unavailable partner in hopes that he would come around and see how special I was, or rather, how special I was to him and that he needed me. It's a pattern I'm still detangling myself from at the age of forty-four. You can probably see how this cycle was shaped by the codependent relationship with my dad.

I was mad at my boyfriend for being that guy. I don't remember the specifics, but I remember he was getting kicked out of school for the intent to deal dope on school property. I stood by him, even though I did not support what he did. I was in a place where it was my turn to feel his support as I dealt with the challenges of college and old childhood wounds coming to the surface. He wasn't there that night when I called, and I was mad. I needed him and he was off in his little world of chaos. So, I went out with my roommates and did what most college kids do when they don't know how to process their emotions and life stuff in a healthy way. I got drunk.

This was a problem for me more so than other kids my age because I had an alcoholic dad and because I already knew I had a problem with alcohol.

I resisted alcohol as a teen because I saw what it did to my dad, and it scared me that I would become that way too. But at the same time, I was never one to feel comfortable with limitations or boundaries. One night, when it felt safe enough at Gabby's house during my sophomore year of high school, I drank, and I got drunk, very drunk. All I remember was that there was a very big bottle of vodka at the beginning of the night, no parents to watch us, her older brother and his cute friend, and the absurd idea that I needed to conquer my fear of alcohol. I remember being slightly tipsy, lightheaded, stumbling, and laughing, and then just like that, lights out. There were moments I regained some level of clarity which consisted of seeing myself being held up by Gabs and her brother above the toilet to make my projectile vomit get in the hole. There were other glimpses of seeing myself screaming and crying hysterically, begging the porcelain gods, "Please don't let me become him!!" or "I don't want this anymore. Please get it out of me."

The next day, I woke up still drunk and my body was sore with fresh bruises all over. The reality I woke up to made me cry again with a deep sense of Shame in who I had become that night. When I went home to Mom's I showered, hid in my bedroom, and tried to sleep off the Shame and Guilt of the night behind me. Thankfully, I had vomited every ounce that was inside of me, leaving me empty, but I am sure I still reeked of the whole experience. I never understood how my mom never noticed or tried to talk to me about it.

I swore to never drink again, and my friends there that night did too, for a while. I seemed to have scared us all straight. I held on to that promise for a few years. But in college I was around it all the time, with friends who looked like they were just having fun. I didn't see the scary ways of my childhood, so I thought perhaps it was safe to try again. I promised myself to be safe. My boyfriend at the time knew about my past and always looked out for me, even though he was somewhat of a bad boy when left to his own devices. He looked out for me, but he wasn't there that night and I had really needed him to be on the other end of that phone.

That is when I chose to drink with my roommates and go to a random house full of guys I didn't know (maybe one of my roommates sort of knew one of them?). It didn't take long for me to get drunk. It was the perfect cocktail for disaster, tiny dancer, mad at a boyfriend, and no real understanding of tolerance of alcohol. Earlier that night, I made eye contact with a somewhat attractive guy across the room because I was mad at my boyfriend for not picking up the phone when he said he would be home. But there I was drunk, my roommates wanted to leave, and I could not move. My eyes and body felt very heavy, I just wanted to take a little nap on the shag rug beneath me and watch the lava lamp drift me into a trance. My roommates didn't put much effort into getting me up and instead asked if I would be okay if they left me there. The guy across the room said he would take care of me. At some point, he managed to get me upstairs into his bed, whether he carried me or walked my stumbling body there, I do not know. While I came in and out of consciousness in his bed, I felt my panties being pulled down off my hips and off each leg. I somehow managed to request that he put a condom on and then lights out again.

I woke up the next morning completely naked with a used condom on the floor next to a pile of my clothes. I got up to pee, grabbed my clothes, and did the walk of Shame before the guy and all his roommates woke up. The smeared mascara and lipstick across my face said everything that needed to be said at seven in the morning, I was a hot mess.

I buried that memory deep inside of me. I would feel the pangs of Shame deep inside my abdomen when it tried to resurface. It only resurfaced once a few months later, when I admitted to my boyfriend that I cheated on him with a one-night stand. It was all so twisted. I felt the guilt of doing something bad; I also wanted to make him feel bad for not being there for me when I needed him, which spiraled me deeper into feeling ashamed for all of it. Despite all that, through Guilt and Shame, he still held me tight as we both wept together on the beach with the morning sun. We stayed together for another year or so and never spoke of that confession again.

I never told my ex-husband because I felt like a whore. I was able to bury the shame inside those fifteen years of our relationship because I vowed to be different.

It resurfaced again after my marriage as I played out the scenario unconsciously with a couple of partners where I allowed them to make me feel Shame again. There was the time I lied to a boyfriend about who I had slept with before, only to tell him the truth later when I knew he would lash out at me and not trust me. There were things that I said to another partner that I knew he would throw back in my face later in disagreements. I somehow wanted to feel those pangs of pain as a reminder that I deserved it all. It finally reared its ugly head a few years ago where I could bring it to the light and see it for what it was. It happened when another high school boyfriend paid me a visit for a weekend reunion. On night one, he got a bit tipsy and told me he still loved me and wanted to make me happy. I held him in my arms and told him that I was not his person, I never felt I was. Even when we were in high school, I felt our relationship was there to get us through something so we could move on through our own lives. I felt like his person was coming soon though and let him know to just hold on a little bit longer. On night two, we both got tipsy, or rather, I got drunk. So drunk that I made a choice that went against every sober ounce of my being. I got up from my bed where we were both lying ready to fall asleep, went to my closet, pulled out a condom, ripped it open with my teeth, and said to him, "You are going to like this." Then lights out. I woke up completely naked on my bathroom floor as he walked in that very moment, threw me over his shoulder, brought me to bed, and just held me.

In the morning, I woke up ashamed. All the pangs of past Shame were like daggers now as we ordered our omelets and awkwardly talked about the night before. I was ashamed that I took advantage of his vulnerability of still pining over me. I was ashamed that I did it so I could have a moment to feel good again; I felt desired. I was ashamed I drank so much I let myself make poor choices. I was ashamed that I let that guy whose name I never even learned come inside of me twenty years earlier.

A few days later, I spilled it all in therapy about the choice I made to take advantage of my friend. My therapist could not quite understand why I was so upset. She saw that I had a night with someone who cared for me, to be intimate with in a safe way. She didn't see the root of it all until I unraveled that night from my past where I made another horrible choice. She paused and said, "Phoebe. Do you know that you were raped?"

I was raped? I had called myself many things about that night but "raped" was never one of them.

Even after that session when those words were uttered to me for the first time to free myself, I still had to deal with the waves of Shame in my own time. It has taken a lot of inner work to look at the pattern that trapped me in the cycles of Guilt and Shame. It still takes a lot for me to look at and share with you on these pages. I even ask myself now, "Is this share necessary?" I ask because maybe, just maybe, sharing this story will make me feel ashamed again and trigger old feelings of unworthiness. But I stop and feel that fist in my abdomen pause, it wants to hold its grip then realizes, no, not anymore. Sharing this story frees me, but my hope—even more so—is that it frees you. I hope to share with you so you can look back at your moments in time/space when you felt guilty, ashamed, and when you made choices to perpetuate those feelings. I hope that fist inside your gut, or wherever it manifests within you, pulls back a little and pauses to give you the space to make a new choice, a new way of experiencing yourself.

I finally traced it all back to that one night, the rainy night I left Dad. When he pushed me out the door without a hug and I thought it was because I was letting him down, and when I sat in the car with Mom, and she didn't hold me to console me. Maybe you, dear Radiant One, already knew it or see it from your vantage point and maybe I always knew too but didn't really believe it: They both loved me but carried their own Shame and Guilt. My dad, guilty and ashamed for the choices he made to put his teenage daughter in a position of leaving behind her family. My mom, guilty and ashamed that she left her daughter behind with a man she didn't feel safe with but somehow thought her little girl would be fine. My mom believed I needed to be there for him and then saw the repercussions of her own inactions. All those years, this moment was trapped in time by all our collective Shame and Guilt.

What began to free us all was one single call on June 21, 2009. My dad called on Father's Day, said he was sober, and wanted to be my father again. It was as if the three of us had held our breath all those years wondering how the choices we made or didn't make would play out in determining how deep the pains of Shame and Guilt would take hold of us for good. With that one sobering call from my dad, eighteen years after that rainy night when it all began, we all exhaled. Over the next seven years, awareness, forgiveness, acceptance, and self-love ultimately freed me from Shame and Guilt's deadly grip.

I no longer seek out situations with alcohol or men to make me feel guilty of my actions or ashamed of myself. I am surrounded by more and more people in my life that see me for who I really am and reflect that radiance back at me, and not those dark, twisted corners of shadows that once haunted me.

The Two Partners, Guilt and Shame, Broken Down

How are they different and how are they partners in crime?

Guilt comes from the actions we take or don't take and the feeling of what comes after. Shame is when we identify ourselves with that action or inaction. In even more simple terms:

Guilt: I did X, so I feel like a bad person.

Shame: I am a bad person who does bad things.

Think of Shame and Guilt as partners in crime because if we don't address the issues of what makes us feel guilty, we become that guilt which then transforms into shame. We no longer tell ourselves we have a choice, but we *become* those choices, and they run our lives. Here's an example: You move from making a few bad choices like eating unhealthy food a few times and then it becomes a habit after life throws you a few curveballs where you find yourself in downward spiral. You then feel guilty about your choices, noticing that your clothes feel tighter, your energy is off or erratic, or your body reacts with poor digestion or some other dis-ease. This is the body's way of signaling that it is simply time to reset. But, if you continue down that road of making those unhealthy choices, Shame steps in and allows you to identify as being "an unhealthy person," "fat," "out of shape," and not worthy of changing your habits.

The deeper I go into exploring the core wound of Guilt and Shame, I see the theme of not feeling seen, heard, or felt in the light that I wished to have been seen, heard, or felt in. I have a feeling the same will be true for you too as I have also witnessed these patterns through my work with others.

As I traced it all back to that rainy night when I left my dad, I wanted him to acknowledge me and tell me I was making the right choice for leaving and not to feel guilty for leaving, no matter what might happen to him. I wanted my mom to hold me and tell me she saw my pain and to help me not carry the weight alone. *Would the outcome have been any different if those two things had happened?* I don't know. I *do* know that these are stories I told myself over the years and told myself because the ways I was not seen, heard, and felt, made me feel unworthy. And, believing that I was unworthy, I kept unconsciously recreating those feelings again and again, as a reminder to feel that Guilt and Shame. It was a vicious circle.

I unconsciously found ways to self-sabotage my relationships so that the men in my life closed the door on me like my dad did on that rainy night. I also found ways to use alcohol as a cry for help which reinforced my belief that people would not acknowledge me in my hour of need. Like when my mom didn't hold me that rainy night or recognize that I reeked of booze when I was hungover from my night at Gabby's. Or my roommates who left me at the party where I was left to get raped and didn't even ask the next day if I was okay. These were just some of the threads.

What I believe is that all our guilt and shame stems from not feeling seen, heard, or felt in the light we wished to have been received in at our core. What I mean by this is we recreate situations where we reinforce that core memory where we first felt those pangs of Guilt and Shame. We begin to tell ourselves these stories, then believe at our core that we are not worthy. We try to take a healthier path but perhaps go in another direction (self-sabotage) that leaves us feeling guilty for those actions that we took or did not take. We identify with the actions or inactions to such an extent that we *become* them (Shame). We say to ourselves, "I am an alcoholic," "I am the one who failed," "I am worthless." We forget the wholeness of ourselves; we become fragmented pieces of ourselves through the lens of Shame. We only see a piece of ourselves that is "bad" versus how that part of ourselves is hurt and wants attention to heal in some way. How does that resonate with you?

The Shameful Twist in the Solar Plexus

We have already explored how the imbalances of our emotions can show up anywhere in the body. My anger and resentment manifested primarily in the sacral chakra, but it may have originated from the uncontrollable fire of anger in the solar plexus. Most texts say that guilt originates in the sacral chakra and when not processed, is transformed into shame which lives in the shadows of the solar plexus.

For our purposes here, we will sit in the solar plexus. This is where I felt my guilt and shame, the tight, twisty fist inside my abdomen, right underneath my diaphragm. It would show up when thinking about those memories and whenever I was on the verge of making a choice I may regret. I started to listen more closely and realized it was cautioning me not to make another move towards self-sabotage that would simply perpetuate the cycle. So, I stopped, and the fist's grip lessened. From then on, I started to make new choices towards expansion and away from the restriction that kept me captive.

A few months ago, I wrote an email to San Diego, about the guilt and shame that I still carried in the role I played within our relationship. A few weeks went by, and he didn't respond. I entered an Akashic Records program and one night, during the course, we planned to go into our records and cut the energetic cord on a relationship that was no longer serving us. I was feeling hesitant, but I knew. I felt like it was time for me to cut the cords for both of us once and for all. I went in and did the ritual I was guided to do; I immediately felt the release of that fist twisted deep inside of me. I had no idea it was still there. I came out of the experience, and we took a break. I went to my phone to check my messages and there was a response from him in my inbox. He said he was sorry too and that we did our best. The grip was gone for both of us. Just like that, Shame and Guilt were free. I haven't felt the pangs and twists of their return in any way since then, thankfully. I did have a small wave after Gabby died but it subsided when I sat in knowing we loved each other. Love and Forgiveness were ultimately my way out of Guilt and Shame every time.

Guilt and Shame may manifest for you as that fist, but it also may land in the body and twist it and wrestle with it somewhere else. I invite you to do your investigation.

Let's Check In

Now let's look at your story. Where do your pangs of Guilt and Shame reside?

First, take a few breaths and sit in the space of my story. What came up for you? Did you feel sensations in your body? Did memories come up? Thoughts? Feelings?

Just sit and breathe for a few moments.

Now, close your eyes and ask yourself:

- When was the first time I didn't feel seen, heard, or felt in the light that I wished to have been received in?

- Sit with that memory for a bit. Go as deeply as it feels safe for you now.

    - Who was there with you? What did they say (or didn't say)? Where were you? What was happening?

    - How did you feel? What were you thinking? What sensations did you feel in your body?

- After feeling, write down anything that comes up for you.

- Did other memories come up when you felt this core memory? Let yourself follow them for a bit.

- Place your hands where you feel a sensation in your body. Allow your hands to feel, see, and hear these memories you have been holding onto. They want to be seen, heard, and felt. Let your hands be a set of eyes, ears, and support for you right now.

- Breathe. Pause. Write. Sit. Witness. Breathe. Pause. Keep repeating until the waves of these memories and feelings move through you.

- You may want to cry, you may want to scream, you may want to do something completely different. Honor it. Whatever comes up, let it flow out. It wants to be seen, heard, and felt without judgment, without feeling guilty, without feeling it has to be something else, without "shoulding" yourself (*you should have made a different choice, you should have acted better, etc.*)

After you let this energy flow through you, calm and self-soothe with the following choice of mantras:

- I am worthy.
- I am seen, I am heard, I am felt.
- I deserve to receive love and to feel loved and to be loved.
- I am whole and complete.
- There are no right or wrong choices, just choices.

After you have soothed yourself. Perform a ritual to release this contract with your core wound. Here are a few ways to go about this:

- Write your letter to Guilt and Shame.
- Write up an agreement or contract with Guilt and Shame, outlining what is no longer acceptable for the roles they play in your life and a promise for you to uphold yours. Please note, these are not "shoulds" that will haunt you in the future. These are clear intentions of what you want to bring into your life and where you want to set your attention, to quiet the noise of Guilt and Shame.
  - Guilt and Shame, you are not allowed to make

me feel unworthy if I don't/do…

- I promise to focus my attention on… to work my way to…

- Let yourself sit in the space of your body and feel what you want to feel without the weight of Guilt and Shame. How does it feel to relax without it? Keep revisiting this feeling to change your sensational patterns.

When those moments that trigger you come up with the inner dialogue of "I should be doing X," or "I didn't do X, so I am Y," or "I am X," pause. Breathe. Come back to the mantra of choice and watch your story begin to shift.

Now, whatever you are feeling in this moment, finish this statement:

As I release Guilt and Shame, my body tells the story of…

Letter to Loneliness and Misunderstood

Dear Loneliness and Misunderstood,

Maybe people don't think of you two being so interwoven at first glance, but I think when it comes down to it, you two are best friends that are directly tied with communication. If we don't know how to communicate efficiently, we feel you both on some level.

Loneliness, we have had a life-long relationship since I was a child, an only child who had to keep secrets and saw the world differently from others. You and I spent a lot of time together, even into my adulthood during my marriage. I am convinced that you have fallen in love with me, as you spent years lurking in the shadows and waiting for me to fall into your open arms, into your abyss where you quietly wished for me to stay with you forever.

I think you have fallen so deeply in love with me, that you are now in cahoots with Misunderstood, to make sure that others don't get close to me. You want us to be together forever, and most recently, I must admit that I am beginning to surrender to this idea. I don't mind you as much these days since you seem to have transformed into a softer and gentler version of yourself. A version that some might call by a different name—Alone. In our time and space together, we have spent it writing these words, dancing, crying, laughing, walking in nature, traveling, and so much more. You have become my most intimate partner. You know everything about me, and you still don't go away.

The first time I felt your presence was that night Mom left Dad and the two of us sat together outside watching the fireflies. I watched them fly away just like all the memories of Mom, Dad, and me that would be no longer. They were all leaving me, but you were there holding my little hand and got me up for school the next day to face my new life. I would feel you the following years when I danced with you, not knowing it was you. I felt a presence, it was almost like someone was watching me from my window, or at least that was what I wished because I wanted someone to notice me. I look back now and think that must have been you.

I am surrendering more to this idea that perhaps you are the one I have been searching for this whole time. You have always been there for me when no one else was. You somehow kept me safe the nights I wished that I would not wake up the next day, when I cried out for someone, anyone, to hear me and see me, you were always there. So maybe it is time to lean back and fall into your abyss and let the rest of the world figure it out for themselves as we dance together for eternity. Would anyone even notice?

Misunderstood, you sometimes brought conflict with others (and I think more so as you and Loneliness decided to pair together) but mostly it was the conflict within myself. I didn't often get in fights or misunderstandings with friends or partners (more on that soon) but I found myself having to hold back my words to protect Dad or Mom, to protect what other people thought of me or my family, or simply because I could not find the right words to express myself to someone else. I also became afraid to use my words because I thought I would push people away. To protect myself from being rejected, I stopped saying what I felt for a while.

Being you, Misunderstood, was familiar to me because the movement was my way of communicating and not many people in my world knew how to communicate like that. I understood others and their words to some extent (not necessarily the choices in how they thought to see the world), but I never felt they got me or took the time to know my way of seeing and experiencing the world. I would say things and hear them recall the same message but to someone else's credit days, weeks, or years later and I would say, "I already saw that and said that!" For this reason, you and Loneliness worked together to isolate me from others.

You both were in my marriage. Neither my husband nor I enjoyed conflict, so you both sat in the silence and distance between the two of us. I don't know exactly what happened but somehow what little voice I did have became smaller and smaller in that relationship. After our divorce, Anger showed up with the two of you and I began to speak up in a tone that was often directed at the wrong person. Fear was there too, as I was afraid of trusting and falling in love with someone so the two of you thought perhaps it would be easiest to just be with you both. I could hang out with Misunderstood and Loneliness, and not have to deal with the Anger, Fear, and Grief again. You both were protecting me, I guess.

We have been negotiating a lot over the last few years though, which I am very grateful for. Still, I have found myself having to part ways with people who do not understand my intention or words. Fortunately, I have found my way to be okay with that. Misunderstood, I hope to see you less and less but know you will always be around for those who are not ready for what I have to say. I am standing my ground and speaking up when I feel it is necessary and stepping away when it becomes toxic on any side so that I can use my energy more efficiently for the people who do understand me. Loneliness, when I have to part ways with people, you send a pang of pain in my heart, but the intensity feels a bit less than in the past.

Because of the lessons with the two of you, I am learning how to communicate better, especially when I need to stand my ground or when I need to listen and be more receptive. None of us are perfect, so Forgiveness and Acceptance usually follow behind you now to help bring clarity to the space.

I want to also say thank you for bringing me closer to my other great love, Dance. You two tightened our bond over my life and have always allowed me to flow freely with it when no one else was looking or listening. You were both necessary for me to get to where I am now, to help others who feel your presence too so that I can better understand what they feel, hold their hands, and let them know they are seen, heard, and felt. It seems to be a very necessary journey to spend with you so I can better serve our world.

With grace,

Phoebe

Layers of Loneliness

There are so many reasons that bonded me with Loneliness. To start, I was an only child for the better part of my childhood. I had an older half-brother who I'd never met before he died in a motorcycle accident. I also had an older half-sister who I didn't know about until I was older and then, barely spent time with her. We parted ways when my dad died because it was just too complicated for me to carry on any kind of relationship with that side of the family. Both siblings were from my dad. None of my aunts on my mom's side had kids until I was in high school, and my baby half-sister didn't arrive until I was a senior in high school. So, I spent a lot of time alone when I was with my family. When I received attention, it was usually compromised with either limited time to play with me or negotiating to play a game that only grown-ups liked, like Trivial Pursuit. I have never been someone who enjoys knowing random and trivial facts so playing this game at any age, especially under ten was not fun at all. It was my personal hell.

Most holidays were spent with my mom, aunts, their boyfriends, sometimes my gramma, and my Grandpop Bob in a house that he rented for all of us. There usually wasn't a designated bedroom for me, since I was the youngest and could be put on a pullout couch, in a bed with Gramma, or on couch cushions in the corner of a room. At some point when I felt Misunderstood and Loneliness creep in, I ended up in a corner away from everyone crying quietly to myself because someone ignored me or said something hurtful to me. At the time, I also didn't quite understand that being an empath meant I felt what was not being said among others. I often questioned the emotions that suddenly came *through* me. I felt the best action to take was removing myself from the environment that overwhelmed me. My mom usually broke free from the group and checked in to see if I was okay and pat my back until I would cry myself to sleep. There was one Thanksgiving when Gabby got to come with me on my family vacation which made a world of a difference; we made paper-mâchéé masks and went on adventures exploring the woods together outside.

The other layer of my relationship with Loneliness was living alone with my dad and having to keep secrets as to what was happening in our home: the anger, the rage, the drinking, the drama with his girlfriends, his spending my child support money on drugs, his drug use, his absence, his relapses, his lying to me, and the somewhat veiled threats from his drug dealer. All of that to say, I felt my ability to communicate with others was not authentic in many ways. I couldn't express myself fully to my mom in case she decided to take me away from Dad. I was embarrassed to tell my friends. I never felt truly connected with people, which often left me feeling lonely and misunderstood. I remember when things were really bad, I would go through my list of people I could potentially reach out to: Mom, Gramma, my aunt, Gabby, and yet, I always found an excuse as to why I could not talk to them about any of it.

There was one time that I felt I had my chance, and I blew it. My dad's girlfriend and her college-aged daughter were living with us at the time. Dad was in such a horrible mood and was demanding that I go and pick up sticks in the yard while he did other work outside. I did not want to be anywhere near him and his energy. I kept making excuses about doing housework inside and he kept yelling at me to come outside. I reluctantly came down and started putting on my shoes to do my dreaded chore. He was outside moaning and groaning about something to his girlfriend. Deciding I was not moving fast enough, he grabbed me and threw me across the yard into the pile of sticks, then picked me up and threw me into the trash cans. I saw my neighbor across the street see what was happening. He ran inside and I prayed he would call the cops and get this evil man away from me. Nothing happened that day though; I dusted myself off and did my chore with whimpers.

That evening, his girlfriend's daughter came home and came to my room. She was angry at me because I had been in her room and borrowed her sweatshirt. It was something I was guilty of, but I wanted to look cool like her and wanted to feel seen positively. On her way out, she said her mom told her what happened to me that day. She said that my dad was having a bad reaction to the drugs the VA gave him for his shellshock and that I should understand that it wasn't my fault and not his fault either. It took away any hope of anyone understanding and seeing me. My dad's girlfriend never actually spoke to me about it herself and she ended up moving out a few weeks later after we got veiled death threats on a voice machine from Dad's drug dealer Dwayne, who needed money from him.

A couple of weeks later another neighbor called me to check in. She asked if my dad was okay and if I was okay. She asked if he did anything to hurt me. I had already shut it down and surrendered to the loneliness of not feeling seen at that moment, so I denied it. It was done and I wanted to move on. A week later I was in my counselor's office about something else and she asked me too, informing me that my neighbor had called my school to follow up. I denied it again and felt even more embarrassed that the word might be spreading.

I have looked back at these moments, wondering if I should regret not saying anything then. *What if I had? Would he have gone to jail? Would I have had to change schools to go live with my mom?* Those were my initial thoughts and I just wanted things to stay the same, even if I felt lonely in my choice. But perhaps in some ways, it empowered me to speak up the following year when things started to take a turn for the worse with Dad. I had finally been acknowledged by other people that what he was doing was not okay when he threw me into the sticks and so when he spiraled even further down, I had to speak up. It was uncomfortable and scary, really scary. It is what led me to leave Dad less than a year later which again, I asked myself for eighteen years *did I regret leaving him?* as Guilt and Shame gnawed at me. I wondered if speaking up for myself was worth losing him and feeling Loneliness.

The final layer to Loneliness and Misunderstood is the fact that I have always felt and seen the world differently from others around me. In my family, they talked about politics which I did not understand at all. I saw energy, dance, movement, feelings, and how everything was interconnected through our stories. The conversations around civil rights, abortion, health care, all sounded like obvious points—taking care of everyone, no matter race, ethnicity, and financial status should be a nonissue, and everyone should be free to make choices to live a healthy and happy life. I didn't understand how other people could think otherwise and how we could be arguing over matters such as these. I often thought that humans made up reasons to create conflict and pain.

Even though I was in the dance community at an early age, I still felt a bit separate from them. I had a few dancer friends and we truly supported one another but even there, I didn't quite feel they saw dance as I did. It wasn't until I went to college and had the opportunity to study with Bill T. Jones for a summer in Saratoga Springs, that things shifted. Each student got to have lunch with Bill and ask him anything. A gay, Black man, at least double my age at that time, battling HIV who had lost his partner to AIDS. We had nothing in common on the surface, but we had the language of dance. It was the first time I felt a fellow dancer and respected teacher really saw me, connected with me, and was interested in who I was not just because of how high I leaped or how many turns I could do. We sat there in the cafeteria having the same mediocre pizza from similar blue plastic trays and talked about life. I asked him about having HIV and how he took care of himself daily. He told me that each day was a new opportunity to keep going and to listen to his body to take care of it. I had read his autobiography before I met him, so I knew that he had some years behind him where he was a bit wild with the choices he made with his body, and that resonated with me on a deep unconscious level. We also talked about what it meant to "play the game" in the world of an artist and how it was ultimately up to me if and how I chose to do it. I did not know exactly what that meant yet since I had not formally started my career, but his words stayed with me throughout my city years as a dancer and I carried them with me onto my path as a yoga teacher. At that table, I promised myself and him I'd always move with integrity, whether that was part of the game or not. Within that conversation, he also shared with me his perspective of what balance is: being able to be still in the midst of chaos while being stable and in control and being able to work oppositions and keep them at the same level of intensity.

This conversation will always be cherished, even though it was fleeting. The following years I auditioned for him a few times and he sometimes kept me for callbacks and other times looked right through me like the other choreographers who have stared at a room full of hundreds of dancers for hours on end. I was just out there again in the sea of dancers, hoping to be seen and understood again. When I *was* seen and understood in an audition, rehearsal, or on stage though, it was pure magic.

Being on stage is another layer of feeling Loneliness and Misunderstood. I felt dreadfully alone, particularly when performing solos at times. I can understand how someone who has never been on stage could be perplexed by this, so let me explain. When on stage, the lights shine so brightly on you, you look out to the audience and the wings, but you cannot see beyond the lights. You see darkness on the other side, a darkness that sometimes feels bleak. At times you can make out silhouettes or see the reflection of someone's glasses, and maybe, just maybe you can even see a few bright smiles if you can take a moment to focus out there. I sometimes felt the awe of my movement in the audience's bodies which made me feel connected with them. I felt seen and understood and a vessel for them in some way to express what they might know was possible for themselves. That was pure magic when that happened. But when I could not feel them, I did not know if I was being understood. I did not know if they felt that connection or if it was just me, all alone exposed in the light.

As performers, we often go backstage and report to the other performers about the energy of the audience and if it is "dead." (Did you know you are an active participant in a performance, and we need you to be present with us?) I have had so many visions (and other healers have had the same visions for me) where I begin to dance on a stage, and then the lights come up and the audience dances with me. That is how Mvt109™ came through: to break down the walls of the proscenium stage and lights. This way we can dance together, feel connected, and no longer feel Misunderstood and Loneliness from the separation of the light and dark.

The worst compliment John gave me was, "You were the best in your row." My heart sunk every time he said it. It was an insult and demeaning. It is as if he wasn't even bothering to look at me. He didn't get who I was, what my soul was saying through my movement, what I could not express to him in words. After pouring my heart and soul into a performance, he just brushed me off. It killed a piece of me, every time. After years of putting every ounce of my energy into a performance and not feeling like I was seen or understood I gave up. I wanted to *feel* something. I wanted to know it meant something to someone out there. I even hesitate now as I write this book for you because I am asking the same thing now that I did then, "Will they get it? Will they understand what my message is?"

A few minutes before I wrote this, I came out of a Shamanic journey where my question was, "What am I not seeing to allow my energy to feel reciprocated?" I came out crying with the vision of me again on a stage, looking out into the abyss and pleading, "I want to feel them!" Now I come here to be on a metaphorical stage to help others see themselves. I am surrendering to that now, but I still want to feel you and know you are out there too. I think that is ultimately what we all want for ourselves: to feel seen, heard, and understood.

Our Collective Loneliness

I think there is a Loneliness epidemic in our culture, and it comes from not feeling seen or heard. On some level, we don't feel as understood or connected as we used to when we were a more community-based society. Our Western world can have us feeling isolated and not good enough. In addition, social media has become an integral part of how we connect with others which is detrimental to our mental health and nervous system. We are taught to be individuals yet if we don't do it in a certain way, we are not accepted. I am referring to ways of thinking and seeing the world, leaving the race, ethnicity, gender, sexuality out of it since those conversations are dominant elsewhere (and need to be had during these times). I am intentionally addressing how we each see, move, and live in our world as spiritual beings in any kind of human body. Through all my encounters of teaching, guiding, and just being human with other humans, I continually witness that all of us on some level have experienced not feeling seen, heard, or felt whether it was by the masses, a random stranger, or our mother. We all are living some kind of story of Loneliness and feeling Misunderstood.

We can go into asking the question if society set us up for this isolation, but that could turn into a whole other book. Here, we will sit with how to shift this experience for yourself. How are you going to remember that you have the choice in how you communicate with your world and how you want to feel seen and heard? Maybe you want to have two million followers on TikTok, be a movie star, or maybe you would rather just be seen by the few people that know you and love you. You get to choose, and we will sit with that here in our practices.

Cutthroat With Words

In the energetic body, our throat chakra is usually the place we are blocked when we don't feel we are properly communicating with others in a way we feel seen, heard, or understood. This is not just the throat but our mouth, jaw, ears, and neck. Think about it for a minute, was there a time you had to hold back your words, bite your tongue, lose your voice? Did it manifest into a pain in your jaw (TMJ), a canker sore, or laryngitis?

There was a period in my late teens and early twenties when I was getting chronic strep throat with really big nasty white lesion-like things infiltrating the back of my throat that no one could see unless I cracked open my jaw and had them look at my grossness with a flashlight. This was always followed by a look of disgust on their face. This was a time in my life I was carrying a lot of shame and guilt for leaving my dad, but I didn't feel safe sharing it with anyone or speaking my truth. I kept it inside of me for no one else to see unless I got cracked wide open. I suffered alone, let it fester, and dealt with the infectious thoughts alone.

Our body can be speaking to us on a deeper level until we decode it and understand it. What is your body telling you right now? How are you listening? How are you not listening? Communication starts with listening to your body first. When you feel like you are holding back your words, listen to how your body holds them in; it doesn't have to be just in the throat. It also goes for the receiving end too. When it is hard to accept someone else's truth that is being shared with you, how are you closing yourself and your body off from it? Where do you feel the resistance in your body?

Start to ask your body questions and see how it wants to express your truth. This can be a gateway to opening the channels of communication with yourself and with others so that you can feel more understood and maybe even less lonely.

Let's Check In

Let's first figure out what Loneliness is to you.

How does that feel for you? What does it feel like in your body? What thoughts do you have? What type of emotions comes up with it?

When do you feel triggered?

- Is it when you are all alone and feel you have no one to talk to?

- Is it when you are in a room full of people, and no one knows you are there?

Are there certain people who make you feel like this or don't understand you?

Why do they make you feel this way?

Once you identify the who, what, where, when, and why, let's sit with how you can make the shift.

Here are a few of my favorite practices to feel less lonely and more understood:

For Loneliness, A Friend Who Holds Your Mirror

This year I chose to detangle myself from some relationships that were no longer feeding my soul. I knew that, because I was about to step onto this massive journey of vulnerability by sharing my whole life here with readers who might have their own ideas and opinions about me and judge me, I needed to be surrounded by people who would be my cheerleaders. To feel safe in my vulnerability with you here, I had to feel supported and trust that what I was saying was with the clearest intention and not wrapped up in a dramatic relationship that may steer my ego off course. In that space, I felt massive waves of loneliness and questioned each step. What helped me was calling on two friends, a woman who is my best friend and a man who is a new friend but with whom I share a strong connection. I told them both that if I texted, "I need to feel supported" to write back how they appreciated me and our relationship. I only had to do this a few times, but each time I did, they wrote me an extremely long text to show me that I was seen, heard, felt, understood, and appreciated. It was what I needed for both my ego and my soul to feel connected again and to remember our collective desires of wanting to be seen, heard, and felt. I always followed it up with gratitude for their message and returned the gift by letting them know how much they mean to me, which turned out to be what they needed too! It's magic to look in the mirror of the people we love and see a reflection of deep appreciation, love, and gratitude. Now, you try it!

- Reach out to a couple of friends (at least two people in case one is unavailable during your loneliness meltdown). Let them know they will be added to your "reach-out" list and what you need from them if you text, call, or email and say, "I need to be seen, heard, and felt!" Or whatever words resonate with you.

- Ask them to respond with a list of why they are grateful for who you are in this world.

- Then, when those waves come up, reach out and trust they will reflect exactly what you need (and I guarantee it will probably be even more because you are that freakin 'awesome!).

- Make sure you respond to them in a way that is sincere and authentic. Trust me, when the tears well up in your eyes from reading their words, you will naturally respond with love for them right back! Take this a step further to spread the love and just send them an appreciation text when they least expect it.

For Feeling Misunderstood, Say It Out Loud and Express Yourself!

When no one seems to be listening or the someone that is supposed to be listening is not, make sure you still get your words out, so they don't get trapped in your body or become something else like resentment. Saying them out loud does not necessarily have to be saying it with your mouth. Instead, this could be writing an angry journal entry with a heavy weighted hand, so the pen pierces through on to the next page to leave an indentation and the paper feels the power of your words. Or, it could be dancing to a sad, lonely song, or singing a musical number you know by heart at the top of your lungs, imagining you are on Broadway and all eyes are on you and your next move.

Write a Letter

Sometimes it does not have to be your literal words you need to get out, and sometimes it does. Listen to what is necessary and how your body needs to process it. My favorite thing to do when I have words to say to someone and I don't feel they are listening to me is to write a letter without a filter. If you plan to send it, take a day away from the first draft and go back. Make sure it still feels necessary and do a few thoughtful edits if that feels good to you. I also support sending it raw (but again, just give it a day to make sure it is still your truth). I used to live by "You can't say the wrong thing to the right person." I still believe it, but I think I tested my limits a bit too much during the angry and fearful stages of my life. If that person is meant to be in your life, they will truly see you for who you are, deeply understand where you are coming from, and hopefully, still be open to communicating. Ask before you send it, "If this person does not receive it in the way I hope they do, will I be okay with that?" If the answer is yes in your body (I usually feel an ease in my belly), then go for it.

If you don't plan to send it, then let yourself fully see it, hear it, feel it. Notice as you read it, how your body feels. Is there a rush of intensity to read your truth? What does that feel like? Read it over and over again, out loud even, and maybe even to a supportive friend, until you don't feel the charge in your body anymore. Let the energy roll through you. Burn the letter, bury it, let your words be taken by the ether or earth to be transformed into something new for you.

After you have given your words up in a ceremony, ask yourself, "What do I need to know to feel understood by this person?" Listen. Deeply listen to see what comes up, and then move from there. Trust that you will be heard by this person or that person may just step away to make space for someone else who will value you, see you, hear you, feel you, and make every effort to understand you because YOU deserve that!

Transforming Loneliness to Being Alone

What I came to realize about Loneliness is that it is focused on our connections, or lack thereof, rather than focused on celebrating you, wanting to be with yourself, and actually enjoying the presence of being with yourself. If you don't want to hang out with yourself, who else will?

Now, try not to go down the self-pity path with this one. Stay here with me.

A friend said to me last night that he is currently "enabling his interests." I perked up with this idea. He said that he made a list of all the things he enjoys or is curious about and allots time during his weekend to discover them more, alone.

I loved this idea because I have been guilty of "waiting for the partner" to come along to enjoy things with. This past summer my mantra was, "No more waiting." I have been making choices like my friend to "enable my interests" on my own and I have been loving it!

- To start, make a list of all the things you enjoy doing, learning about, and/or are curious about.

- Do a little research and see what is possible for you. If it is something you want to do but lack friends or other loved ones to go along with your interest enabling, join a class or a meetup group where there are like-minded people (Yes! you can be alone within a group and not feel lonely!).

- Schedule time for you. In my chapter about Joy, I will guide you through my Unstructured Playtime for Joy so you can carve out the time and space to do it alone.

- You can start small but start somewhere. I have a feeling you might enjoy being alone more with yourself, even if you are extroverted like some of my friends. I have a very dear friend who loves being with people and she is the life of the party but travels for work alone a lot. When she travels, she is always on the move discovering places to eat and paths to hike; she enables her interests freely with such a zest for life!

Now, whatever you are feeling in this moment, finish this statement:

As I begin to listen to the messages of my body, Loneliness and Misunderstood begin to quiet down so my body tells the story of...

Letter to Shock and Numbness

Dear Shock and Numbness,

I first ironically felt you, or lack thereof, on that dreadful cleaning day with Mom and Dad. It all happened so fast, and I remember feeling nothing much of it as I inhaled the cloud of pot smoke that encapsulated me at Dad's friend Jim's place. The smoke seemed to take conscious steps to calm his nerves after he passed the gun off to Jim and said, "Man, I almost used this today." I just stood there feeling nothing and looking perplexed as if he had just passed Jim a cucumber. It made no sense in that time and space, and what could have happened if he had chosen to use it didn't really hit me until much later in my twenties when the memory resurfaced in a dream, and I woke up crying.

Numbness, you became more familiar when Dad was getting worse with his lies. They were so obvious and blatant that I was sincerely shocked no one else could see how desperate the situation had become, how seriously unstable my dad had become. Those times he would ask Mom for my child support money in cash so he could go grocery shopping that night but then immediately left me with empty cupboards to go buy his next high with my caretaking money. How could Mom not see the desperation in his eyes and how could he look at me when he knew I would have to fend for myself and say nothing? I said nothing and felt nothing. If no one else cared, why should I have to? I started to check out from my own basic needs for a little while.

You both enveloped me, and Dad's words meant nothing to me; they were hollow. Even the nice words directed to me, I no longer believed. He would say I was incredible and that I could be whatever I wanted to be, and I would be a star if that is what I chose for myself, yet he didn't show up to any of my shows. When I was Sandy in Grease, or captain of poms, or performing a solo in my dance company performances, he never showed up. How could I believe that he saw me as a star when he didn't even come to see me in my actual element? I shut down and became you, Numb. When he said he loved me, I ignored him and changed the subject as if he didn't say anything at all.

You both have come in waves throughout my life, but luckily you don't stay too long when you do. I am grateful to have made choices in my new life that don't call me into a state of using you both as protection. I am a highly sensitive being who wants to feel my way through life. I am grateful for your protection over the years. I understand why you helped me. Thank you for allowing me the space to reflect on the absence of feeling so I can fully, consciously say yes to living more deeply.

I know you have quite a grip on some people, so much so they have become addicted to you through opioids, and other substances to become closer to you, Numbness. I witnessed it through Dad and John, and I see how you can create a seemingly bottomless pit for so many. I am so very grateful I had a rope for my escape to feel my way back.

With love,

Phoebe

Comfortably Numb

There are days in the city that you forget it's the big bad city and everything clicks, runs smoothly, and feels peaceful. You might get a chance to walk through a city park and receive a breath of somewhat fresh air, hear birds sing their morning songs, see smiles or glances from a passerby that feels like they saw you, and *everything feels just right.*

That was my morning as I walked to my chiropractor. It all felt somewhat divine. It was time for an adjustment to keep my body aligned and pain-free from all the harsh pounding on the literal and metaphorical pavement I was doing as a dancer in the city. It was the beginning of September. Earlier that summer, I left my waitressing gig to declare to the world and myself that I was going to make it as a dancer. No more serving overpriced pasta to the pre-theater dinner animals!

Two months before, I had spent July in Italy dancing with a choreographer and had a couple of solos in an evening performance under the stars of Urbino, Italy. I remember how perfect that night was as I held my arms out and walked with the ensemble in a circle to spiral down to the ground and lie there for a moment before continuing with the piece. I took a breath from the stars and said, "I have arrived." It was electric that night. Each piece is woven into the next from an intense flamenco duet to a joyful African trio, and a string of modern and contemporary pieces that told stories of passion, heartbreak, pain, and enlightenment with still an underlying softness of life.

After that performance, I received a handwritten letter from an audience member telling me how that performance made an impact on him. He was a famous Italian writer who told me I had a gift. This letter carried me back to the city with grace and gave me confidence that I would be able to make it as a dancer.

I didn't have the dream dance company gig yet but felt in my bones that I was on my way. What I did have was a full schedule of teaching dance in New Jersey and Brooklyn to kids and teens. It was something closer to what I wanted and way better than serving enormous plates of spaghetti and meatballs to the bridge and tunnel crowd.

My new full-time teaching gig was to begin that September day, so I walked to my chiropractor that morning with a slight pep in my step knowing I was on my way to getting aligned in my body and with my dream. It was a morning that felt like a new beginning.

The August heat, which was held in the concrete buildings during the day and then released through angry hot air gasps at night (which somehow made them more unbearable than the days) had lifted. There was a gentle soft shift in the air, from the smell of urine to the hint of a scent of changing leaves noting autumn was arriving soon. I walked along Central Park as long as I could from West 101st to West 94th and then crossed over the busier streets of Columbus, Amsterdam, Broadway, and my final destination, Riverside. Things seemed calmer than usual. No heavy traffic, no loud horns, a few car radios playing in the vans of maintenance workers that I didn't pay much attention to. I was fully immersed in the first feeling of autumn and what it was about to bring me.

John had just left for a fall tour the day before on a Monday. I would be on my own for about six weeks, which felt good, to find my groove in this new life I had just declared for myself. No more late nights of work with drinks after my shift that left me too tired and sometimes hungover to take a class or an audition the next day. It was a vicious cycle that only gave me two or three days to be productive as a dancer that I was ready to break. This first full day on my own was the start of that new life. I would start with my alignment session and would head out to my teaching gig in New Jersey in the afternoon through the late evening, to then find my way back to the city around 9:00 p.m., way more reasonable than ending my day at 1:00 a.m.

I had left early enough for my chiropractic appointment so I would not feel rushed walking. I finally arrived at his building. The doorman wasn't there to nod me in, so I walked myself to the elevator and went upstairs to his office apartment. I was a few minutes early and let myself into the waiting room, thinking there would be a person or two waiting ahead of me. No one was there, not even his assistant who usually signed me in. Instead, it was quiet with the TV on in the corner which I had never noticed before. It was muted but the image I saw caught my attention. I stopped to watch it and questioned why he would have a movie like *Die Hard* on at 9:00 a.m. for his patients. I just stood in front of it and stared at it quite in awe. The phone rang and out of the bathroom, pulling up his pants, came my chiropractor. We locked eyes; he looked a little embarrassed, but I didn't quite connect it all because I was still trying to figure out what I was watching on the TV screen. It was all kind of slow-motion from there. He answered the phone, canceled the appointment for the person on the other end and hung up the phone. I'm not sure what he said to me after that, but it was about how what I was watching was happening in our city right now, just on the south end of our tiny island that felt like my entire universe. I was confused. I didn't quite get it. He took me into his treatment room, and I lay down on the table. He was always a bit awkward with conversation and today seemed no different. He asked if I had anyone at home and what my plans were for the day. I told him my boyfriend was in LA for the beginning of his USA tour for the fall and I would be heading out to teach my students in New Jersey around 3:00 p.m. He responded that probably wasn't going to happen. He said, "The whole world has changed now." It still didn't quite sink in.

I wrote him a check which he didn't take, and he told me to rest, be safe, and go home. I walked back without the pep in my step that I had just had a half-hour before but instead, I walked very slowly and completely stunned. It felt like my body was walking but the rest of me was somewhere else and I wasn't sure yet where or how to even go about looking for it. The car radios were still on and now I heard the words *Twin Towers, airplanes, fires,* and then I began to hear the sirens off in the distance. *Did I not hear them before?* They were all congregating at the one place we had just seen on TV, the place where two airplanes crashed into the buildings, the images shown repeatedly on a horror reel replay.

I went to the grocery store around the corner from my apartment. This was a place I didn't generally choose to make eye contact with people but as we all made our way through the very tiny aisles gathering our canned food and toilet paper for this apocalyptic moment in time, we all saw each other. We all asked with our eyes if we were going to be okay: tall, strong Black men, little Latino women, and a few white, ghostly looking people. I ran into a fellow dance acquaintance who also knew a couple of mutual friends who were supposed to be dancing that evening with a company at the gardens in the Twin Towers. We wondered if they had been down there for a tech rehearsal. We accounted for all our other people and no one else we knew should have been down there. We gave each other a very meaningful hug, a hug we would have no other reason to share in previous meetings, and went on our way, back into the panicked daze we were all in.

I got home and tried to log on to my dial-up. After a long time, I saw a few emails from my mom who was panicking asking where I was and if I was okay. She told me to call her because she could not get through to me on the phone. I didn't even think about how the rest of the world knew what was happening on my island. I tried to call but had no luck. Lines were busy no matter what number I tried to dial. I couldn't email her because I kept getting kicked off my dial-up. Somehow at some point later that day we got through and she sounded relieved to hear I was okay. There would have been no reason to her (or my) knowledge that I would have been in the financial district at morning rush hour, but she was feeling a lot better knowing I was safe. She then worried about what I was going to do if another attack was coming and begged me to stay home. I did.

All bridges and tunnels were closed, I was not able to go to my teaching gig. I spoke with the dance studio owner, and she reassured me that classes would not be happening that day or perhaps for several days. I received another call from my old restaurant gig in Times Square begging me to come into work that night since they were short-staffed. I said there was no way I would leave my seemingly safe home on the Upper Westside to go to another potential target and hung up the phone. I turned on my TV, adjusted the bunny ears, and sat there in the glow day and night probably for a good week. I did make it to Central Park once or twice that week when I finally felt it was safe to come out of my overstimulating media cave. I met up with Gabby who had just arrived in the city a few months prior and was staying at her uncle's place just a few blocks away. We sat on a park bench smelling the air that reeked of death. There was no other way to describe it. We watched children play as if nothing had changed in their little universes, with a backdrop of missing persons pictures plastered on lamp posts and street signs. There were candles lit for memorials on some corners with a picture of a loved one. Sad, confused, and heartbroken looks in all our eyes, and still the children played. They shrieked with joy as we shared stories heard from friends or from the news about the bodies that were seen leaping from buildings, the images of hundreds of people fleeing through the chaotic streets, just running away, not knowing what or where "away" was.

We didn't see those images firsthand, but we felt them in our city bones. We felt the grief of the lost loved ones, the missing wives and husbands who hadn't come home yet. Maybe they were in a hospital, maybe they were hiding in a dark corner out of sight for the next round of attacks, maybe they found a safe place and just couldn't call home yet, maybe they used this as the opportunity to get out of a life they no longer knew how to live. All the stories that were on our tiny island were being watched and felt around the world. I felt it all within me, yet I was completely numb. I felt numb for a few good years. Journal entry after journey entry I kept inquiring why I felt so numb.

Was it this particular moment in time or was it the general overstimulation of the city that somehow separated my soul from my body, depriving me of my sensational experience of life? It wasn't until perhaps the summer of 2004, a few months before I got engaged, that I started to shift out of the numbness and began to feel myself again.

Shocked to Numb

Shock is something that we all can experience after a traumatic event. I felt this same sense of shock for periods after the traumatic encounters with my dad as a child, and for a while after his disappearance when I was a teenager, and again for several months after his death and during my divorce.

Our bodies and our minds want to protect us but what happens is that in the process we may lose connection to the sensations in our bodies, connections with other people in our lives, and our connection to spirit if we let things go too far. During a traumatic event, our amygdala in the brain can take us "offline" to survive during an event. This is a way of protection. As I learn more about Shamanism, this is also what is called "soul loss" where the soul may leave the body as a way of protection. When the event is over, there might not be a full recovery of returning to the present experience unless there is a full integration again of mind, body, and spirit. If we do not fully consciously integrate and do not address the stress of the trauma over time, one direction we may end up in is a hypo-arousal state of not feeling: physically, emotionally, spiritually, and/or mentally. This could be experienced as not feeling sensations in the body, feeling numb emotionally, not feeling connected to faith as you once had before, or forgetting moments in time from the event or around it.

Aside from this, we may choose to numb ourselves consciously or unconsciously on our own through drinking and drugs (like pain killers) or we may try to feel again by drinking and drugs (like stimulants). Unfortunately, this story we know all too well in our Western world. It is our coping mechanism of choice: using avoidance or putting a quick band-aid on to feel better or to feel nothing at all.

I felt the numbness settle in again in 2008 for a period when John was numbing himself with his painkiller addiction for reasons that are private to him, and as a by-product, I felt nothing because I did not know how to have my empathetic boundaries set for myself. I remember feeling the waves of his numbness overtake me when I entered the door some days. I didn't understand this shift then, but I see it clearly now. This is also a period of my life where I was having lots of dreams that were trying to tell me things: messages I wasn't ready for, that John was disconnected, that I was disconnected, and that we were disconnected from each other. As I look back now, I see how my intuition was screaming at me to pay attention, but I felt nothing.

Whatever brings you to a place of experiencing numbness may have long-lasting side effects when not looked at, like discord in relationships, lack of purpose, depression, and apathy. If you experienced a traumatic event or feel you might have experienced trauma that you haven't been able to acknowledge, I highly suggest seeing a professional, someone who can see you and hear you, who can offer specific guidance for you and your situation.

Let's Check In

Let's use my example:

Where were you during 9/11? This is a question I still get asked twenty-plus years later. I have a feeling we will keep asking each other this for a long time. And now, there is another marker in our collective lives, we ask each other, "Where were you when we went into lockdown?" We may have a memory of it, we may have feelings around it. Take a moment and check in. If you were too young to reach back to 2001, focus on the lockdown of 2020, or another time that we all collectively felt the waves of shock. Do you remember where you were when reality sunk in? Can you remember who you were with? What space were you in? Any sounds, smells, textures of the space? What did the energy feel like at that moment? How did your body respond? Was there a moment of not feeling? Of disconnection?

Amazingly, these two events in our somewhat-recent lives were moments when we all received the news in real time, no matter where we were in the world. Because of the internet, news traveled quickly, which had never happened before. I was shocked that day that my mom in West Virginia knew something happened in NY, just a couple miles from where I lived, and that airports around the world shut down in a matter of minutes on that day over twenty years ago.

We all felt something when we watched the lockdown close in on us. It might have been fear, dread, anxiety, uncertainty, and a whole bunch of other feelings that felt quite intense. We were all feeling something, yet we may have felt like time slowed down and that we were somewhat out of our body as we tried to make sense of the new reality being thrust upon all of us collectively.

So where do we go from here? We acknowledge it. We give it a name. We give it expression before it shuts down our systems to the point of not feeling. These are two universal examples, but you can dig around in your own personal life. Is there a moment in time that you remember *not feeling*, or maybe chose not to feel? Be gentle with yourself as you explore. You don't need to know the reason right now; in fact, you might not be ready to, and I highly recommend seeking a professional to work with when you are ready. Just explore what is here for you now.

Third Eye Looks Inward

Connecting in again with the chakra system, we sit with what we call our third eye chakra. This is located just above our brow and includes the brain, pineal gland, and eyes.

This is where we connect with our intuition, our inner voice. This is the voice that speaks to us in those quiet moments, as protection, guidance, and love. It is the voice I began to shut out because I thought its warnings to keep me safe was a curse. It is that deep sense of knowing, sensing, and feeling. This is where we tap into our "clair abilities."

Clair abilities are like our own superpowers of intuition. They are how we receive these gut instincts, or our inner knowing, that we call our inner voice. There are five abilities to tap into. The best known is clairvoyance, which is seeing visions of the past, present, or future that can help bring clarity to a situation. The other four are clairaudience using the sense of hearing of sounds or voices, clairsentience that is a deep sense of feeling, clairalience connecting with the sense of smell, clairgustance connecting with the sense of taste, and claircognizance is that sense of knowing things we would not logically have known otherwise. We all have these gifts, and some more than others know about them and tap more deeply into them. My hope in some way is for you to tap into yours through these stories and practices.

What is strongest for me is clairsentience, a deep sense of feeling. As you read through my stories you may have seen how my body was sensing things and I didn't always listen. As you read here, have you felt goosebumps when you felt deeply connected with my words? Along the way though, in the expanded awareness practices, you may also have seen visions, heard voices, or a deep sense of just knowing something to be true. This is you tapping into your intuition again and we will continue to play with this feeling throughout the rest of the journey we are on together in this book.

These moments when we cannot feel, when we are in shock or numb, we can call in our intuition and ask for guidance. Sometimes I ask intuition questions like:

What am I not seeing right now?

What do I need to feel connected again?

What do I need to know?

What will help me to feel connected to my surroundings and people now?

You can make your list right now if there is an aspect of your life that you feel you have not put much awareness into lately.

Here are a few exercises that may help you feel again:

If you are feeling numb in your body:

- I have a client who, when she feels anxious, loses the

connection to her feet and legs. If this is you, or there is somewhere else in your body that you feel disconnected from, try this:

- Rub and/or hug your feet/legs as you focus on your breath.

- Notice the connection of your hands to your feet/legs:

    - The texture of your skin or clothing

    - The temperature of your skin

    - The weight of your hands on your feet/legs

- If you can't experience any kind of sensation, let it go; don't try to force it. Instead, try a mantra: "I am okay to feel what I feel now."

- Stay with this for five to ten breaths or however long feels safe for you.

If you are feeling numb in your surroundings:

- Try this if you can't feel connected to your surroundings. This will help you remember in your body how you are present and supported to feel safe again. Begin to integrate it into your daily practice to use if you ever find yourself in those moments of disconnection.

    - Identify supportive surroundings (i.e., chair and/or floor). Connect feet and/or hands to it for five to ten breaths. Notice anything else that is supporting you in the experience like your breath, your senses, any energy that is in your space.

If you are feeling numb emotionally:

- Maybe you feel like you "should be" experiencing a feeling because everyone else around you is. First of all, it is okay if you are not feeling what others feel, but if you are curious, you may want to ask yourself why. Try this journal exercise:

    - Take a few moments to set up a quiet space where you can center and reflect. Keep a piece of paper or your journal and pen near you.

    - Close your eyes if you feel safe to do so and take a few cleansing breaths. Notice if your body responds to your intention to center.

    - Allow yourself to get to a place where you can quiet your mind. You may need to move your body around a little bit if you feel restless. Once you feel more settled, write the following prompts on paper, and let your responses flow without judging or analyzing yourself:

        - What I am not feeling now is…

        - Why I think I am supposed to feel this is because…

        - The sensations in my body right now feel like… (try to stay away from good/bad, pleasurable/painful… Get descriptive)

        - If I had to put emotion to the name of this sensation it would be…

        - I have felt this sensation in my body before when…

        - This sensation I feel now, I want to

release/or want more of because...

If you are feeling numb in your life:

- Many times, when I wasn't sure what to do with my life, I felt disconnected from people, my purpose, my motivation. Here are a couple of ways to tap into the messages from the Universe that might help you get back on the path to your own story:

  - Keep a journal by your bed and as you wake (before you look at your phone) write down dreams and any waking visions, messages that are coming in. Do this for at least a week and look back to see if there was anything you are curious about and would like to follow.

  - Ask a question and pull oracle cards. Notice any signs that light you up again. Follow the breadcrumbs of these messages with curiosity. Don't worry about having to figure it out or getting an answer, just sit in the space of unfolding.

  - Start to pay attention to anything even slightly out of the ordinary, to pull you back into your life. Write them down, notice if there are any patterns. Follow again with curiosity.

Now, whatever you are feeling in this moment, finish this statement:

As I find my way to feeling again, my body tells the story of...

Letter to Chaos and Anxiety

Dear Chaos and Anxiety,

When I was a child, Chaos, you and I were like two peas in a pod. You were what I called "Fun" like those times when Dad would wake me up in the middle of the night because he had the munchies and take me on an adventure. We would drive forty-five minutes from Rockville into Georgetown to get Frankly Fries and socialize with drunk college kids of all kinds. They always thought Dad was "way-cool" and I was a novelty.

There were the other nights we stayed more local when Dad wanted to be more of a social drunk, and he took me to the bar with a dance floor so I could keep busy dancing with the other drunk grownups. We got away with it for a little while, I think the DJs liked me because I got people dancing but then the managers caught on to how popular I was and saw me as a liability. A couple of times after I went there, they made a rule (with a sign and everything) that no one under twenty-one was permitted on the dance floor. So that ended it for us. Looking back, I wonder how these same managers and bartenders who made these rules, still allowed my drunk ass Dad to get in a car and drive us both home. We got pulled over so many times when Dad told me to place the paper bag of opened booze under my seat and to not say anything.

When fun nights were spent at home with you, Chaos, Dad would turn the music up at all hours of the night and he let me sing and dance around the living room. He often gave me soulful talks about how I could be whatever I wanted to be and to never let anyone ever tell me otherwise, and if they did, I had to tell them to "go fuck themselves." He also told me if anyone ever touched me in a way that didn't feel good to "kick them in the balls" and to come tell him so he could go "beat their ass." Ah, those were the fun days with you and Dad, Chaos.

There were also scary times with you, Chaos. These were the times when you introduced me to Anxiety. These were moments where everything seemed to quickly shift to the two of you, Chaos and Anxiety, being the two peas in a pod to leave me experiencing you both on such a deep and frightening level. You both were there on the cleaning day when Dad almost killed Mom during his flashback of Vietnam. There were so many other times when everything felt so peaceful and then out of nowhere, a tornado of the two of you swept right through my life, like the Christmas party when Dad beat Katie inches away from me, when he threw me into the pile of sticks and the walls. The irony of Dad being the one whose own ass he needed to kick for me in those times, was never lost on me. Then there were the many times when Dad left in the middle of the night, and I wondered if he would make it back home. All those times, I just dealt with you, Chaos.

Those scarier times somehow became comfortable to me though, they were well-grooved patterns that had me searching for you through other chaotic adventures within my romantic relationships with men. My high school boyfriend, my first love, would take me on adventures while he drove high and drunk, and just like my childhood, I sat sober in the passenger seat with eyes wide open to see what kind of excitement would unfold for us that night. We met different people outside of our circle of friends at school, heard great music, ended up in random places in the city or the country, made love in the backseat of the car or on the lawn of someone's house, in a public bathroom, on the beach at night, or anywhere where we could possibly get caught. Those were our fun times together with you, and we also had our dramatic moments too, but without the violence I experienced with Dad. My boyfriend and I would get into explosive fights, and he would leave me alone crying hysterically, unable to breathe.

I also found you on my adventures in college and living in the city with John. We had many times that were so tightly wrapped in the arms of you both, Chaos and Anxiety. Many times, when he left me all alone and told me to call Mom because he could not handle how you, Anxiety, held your grip on me with the crying; it overwhelmed him and turned on his "flight" switch. He would tell me I was crazy and needed help. He left me out in the cold on one of the most biting cold nights of the winter. There was a warning not to be outside for more than ten minutes because of the wind chill factor. He left me outside, thirty blocks away from our apartment with no cash or phone that was charged, and he got in a cab to go home. It was a full moon and it called me to the river. I was bundled up and tears froze on my face the moment they left my eyes. Doormen came out of their warm, fancy apartment buildings to ask if I needed them to catch me a cab. I just walked and cried to the moon. I began to walk to that full moon as it hovered over the Hudson River. It seemed to just be on the other side of it in New Jersey, waiting for me to come be with it for eternity. It taunted me and begged me to swim to it. I walked to the river, cried out for an answer; I considered making that leap because being in my skin was just too unbearable, but I didn't. A quiet voice broke through the Chaos and Anxiety and whispered to stay still and get some rest. I turned down your voices that were masked as my dear friend the Moon and went home. When I got to my apartment, John was asleep. I sat in the hallway and asked to release you both now that I was home safe. My body shook uncontrollably, I wept horribly loudly, and struggled to reclaim my breath again. I started to feel the warmth of my body return to normal. I called Gabby and she helped me find my center again. She was always there. I can still hear her voice, "Pheeebs, what's wrong?"

During this period of marriage, Anxiety, you seemed to have a daily grip on us, it's like you were a virus that we passed back and forth to each other. John would have more anxiety attacks that I felt on such a deep, intense level that somehow, I manifested into my own. He resented me for feeling his pain like he wanted to be the only one to feel it. Whenever I felt any pain, he claimed I was upset for no reason but when he felt it, he got medications and diagnoses that perhaps validated him.

After my divorce, it was just me to figure out what kind of hold you both had on me without anyone else's energy around to pick up. It's been an eight-year journey of bringing all your influences into my awareness in the roles you both played throughout my life.

There were a few years I recognized you but still decided to choose you, Chaos in disguise as Passion and Excitement in the beginning stages of falling in love again and running my own business with no parameters like I was in the wild west. I got exhausted by the two of you though and decided to call it quits again. It is still a process detangling from you both. I see how I want to lean into the man who may bring in just a little bit of Chaos into my life again (oh just a little bit won't hurt, right?) and how I could care less about anyone who feels like they could possibly be stable and consistent (aka boring). I am getting better though; I am seeing the pattern and making new conscious choices.

I have come to terms that you both will always be hanging around, just waiting to see if I will come out and play with you again. I see you. You are no longer creeping up on me in the shadows pushing your adventures on me like a drug dealer selling "candy" on the corner. I now at least know you are there. I can choose consciously to walk towards you or let you walk right by me without even a hello. It is all a choice now. I have that power within me. I am proud of myself for making these new choices and new worlds are opening up to me because of it.

So, Chaos, thank you for all our adventures together. I will speak of those "fun" days and hold those memories in my heart fondly but do not see that as an invitation back to come in to destroy what order I have. Anxiety, I am finally beginning to figure you out. You show up in ways that feel a bit different from how others express they experience you. We have a unique relationship. You don't hang around me much as you do with some other people, but when you do, it feels like you come right through the door with Chaos, like a tornado full of tears that leaves me exhausted and feeling isolated and alone to pick up the debris of relationships. I am changing that now. I am starting to make sense of what's real and what lies you are telling me to confuse me, like I am in a snow globe that has been turned around and upside down, and I don't know which way is up. I have found my way out of it with my two feet on the ground again. Something I have also discovered is that sometimes when I think you are near, it is Expansion, since you both feel similar with the frenetic energy that buzzes through my body.

I must come to peace with the fact that you both are always here inviting me to play with you, but I choose how I play your games. Chaos, you can come over for a party, but I am not letting you sleep in my bed anymore.

With love and gratitude,

Phoebe

A Chaotic World

I do know Chaos well. When the world went into lockdown for the pandemic in 2020, it was all so familiar, even though I was on the other side of the world in Bali and never experienced a global pandemic before. While I received anxious messages from friends and family in the States, and read the news blurbs of pandemonium, I even said to myself, "Yeah, I got this." My lifelong relationship with Chaos prepared me. I know how to maneuver through the intensity of chaos well, and as I shared even searched it out, and recently have begun to embrace it more and more.

When I went through my divorce, I detangled and re-tangled with Chaos again and again. It got to a point when I asked my therapist if I was bipolar. After her assurance and years of therapy, I now believe that I am not. It was simply just what I knew. I was conditioned to live in a bipolar world, which somehow made me ready for anything, like a global pandemic.

I found Chaos mainly through people, the energy they brought to the relationship that felt wild, exciting, unpredictable, and spontaneous. But over time, the more aware I became, it felt exhausting, ungrounding, and the unpredictability was predictable, catching me in a loop that ran over and over again.

There have been times though that I felt the anxiety of never getting out of that damned loop to the point I felt I would be locked into the pattern of chaos forever (ironic, right?).

I didn't just search it out in relationships with men but also some friendships with women and through dance. I still believe we need chaos in our lives to be an artist. This is why Chaos and I have always been in a somewhat codependent relationship, which I am recently reclaiming as a co*creative* relationship. Chaos through relationships has been a long and steady process of detox that I now feel grounded in, and I trust that I will stay on that path as long as the awareness and boundaries are held. Chaos and I will always dance together in some way.

As artists, we thrive by seeing and experiencing the creation of the universe through us and our medium to try to make sense of the world for ourselves and our spectators. This is why I have recently allowed Chaos to be my muse and let it move through my vessel as a container for the magic to happen. I do my best with that, but Chaos does not always listen and sometimes has its own agenda. We are finding a space to co-exist.

When I was in Bali in March 2020, the chaos erupted beneath all our feet rather quickly, and I somehow held my ground. Our retreat was the first ten days of March. As the days approached, attendees reached out with apprehension as to whether it would be safe to travel. I assured them they would be safe but to take precautions, whatever that meant for them. I wasn't nervous. I had been traveling the months leading up to it and didn't sense we would be in danger. I trusted everything would be okay for our group. As a retreat leader, I instilled the confidence we all needed to move forward.

We stayed on a property that felt like home for me since I had been there three years prior. Everything felt rather calm in our little protective retreat bubble. The last three days we spent in Ubud, we felt the stirrings and whispers getting louder about COVID. My friend, Meghan who came on the retreat had to leave on March 7th to get back home. Before she left, she shared with me a notification from her job saying that our world might be closed down for at least a year because of the spread of this mysterious virus. We were both in a bit of disbelief but contemplated what life might look like very soon.

It started to feel more real, but I still trusted everything would be okay for our group. By the last night of our retreat, March 9th, we all attended a full moon cacao ceremony on the property where we were staying. You could not resist the buzzing of energy of the cacao, full moon, over one hundred people in ceremony, and the humming news of the virus underneath it all. We all danced around in the space and were invited to hug one another in celebration of life, some people hesitated but did it anyway, others elbow bumped or waved from a distance, and then some others came over with a full sweaty embrace.

Let me pause and make it clear if you have never experienced Bali. It is another world. It is named the Island of the Gods for a very good reason. Everyone seems to float in Bali. Everything is sacred, even the shadows are embraced and accepted for the mystical qualities they bring. Making the choice to fully embrace the experience we were in, was its own beautiful Goddess of Chaos inviting us to play. I hugged everyone in that space that wanted a hug because I knew Chaos well enough by then to know I would be okay; this was the fun adventurous version that loved to play.

The first time I landed in Bali was in 2017 for my first retreat there. The energy of Bali was intense then too and brought out heavy detoxifying emotions for my students. At that point in my life, I did not have healthy boundaries with my students, and to make things more interesting, my gramma was with me, and we shared a room. I had no real space to recover each day. I also did not have a strong enough self-care practice to make sure I was energetically cleansed.

On the last day of the retreat, I broke. I still can't quite tell you what happened, but it seemed to have been a cocktail of all the energy from everyone, my period (which was getting worse each cycle), and some kind of flashback that was triggered within me. I snapped. I had a story in my head that morning and began to cry hysterically, like the lid on my container could not hold the chaos brewing within anymore.

I told the group I could not teach them and ran to my room and wept. My gramma followed me and crawled into bed with me. I kept sobbing and asked, "Why did she leave me?" Gramma asked me who I was talking about. I sobbed back, "Mmmmooooom." I was back in that night when Mom and Dad split up. "Why did she leave me?" My Gramma finally responded, "She didn't leave you, Phoebe. She left your dad." It took many sobs for this to sink in and remember where I was. Everything got quieter, the tornado of Chaos ripped right through and left the debris behind for me to make amends with my students.

It was one of the most humbling moments of my life as a teacher and one of the more frightening moments that I was responsible for as a person. I saw my mother-wound up close and personal right there with Mama Bali, showing me herself. When she calls you to play in your shadows, you must be ready for it. When I returned home, the trajectory of my healing journey took a new direction with deeply healing my relationship with my mom and what I am also beginning to piece together, my healing in relationships with men.

Those two and half years since my visit with Mama Bali brought me to my knees. I spent most of it single in solitude while I made sense of my various relationships, mainly with myself and Chaos. So, upon my return to Bali with the threat of a global pandemic, I felt ready when the full sweaty embrace of Chaos came to me.

COVID was present but I felt I was untouchable like I knew that wasn't part of my dance with Chaos but for others to dance with. My group left the next morning after our sweaty cacao ceremony. I was left alone with one other attendee, an assistant/friend who decided to go on her way for the rest of the trip. We still had another week to rest in the arms of Bali.

That week, rest was about the only thing I was able to do. Each day there were more and more shutdowns of businesses making it harder to do things except write in my little Airbnb in the middle of a rice field and eat delicious dragon fruit and pineapple at the little sanctuary around the corner. I received messages from home that were highly anxious and conflicting: come home; don't come home; you will be better off there; the health care system will crash there, and you will be left to die alone. You know, the kind of messages we were all receiving on some level during a global pandemic.

By March 15th, the world seemed to be in a full-blown state of panic. I decided to host a live meditation on social media to calm whoever showed up. I started to offer evening movement and morning meditations for the Western world to get people back in their bodies to feel safe again and trust that their bodies had the elixir they needed during the states of chaos. I felt it was necessary to show up and be a voice of calm. I felt safe and had purpose in the center of this chaos. I felt I belonged and that belonging had to do with me being in the center of the storm, seemingly safe in Bali.

I contemplated staying until the very last moment I entered the airplane on March 18th with one foot still in a cab ready to rest back in the heavenly rice fields. It was close though. The Universe asked me if that's what I wanted the whole way home. When I arrived at the Bali airport, there was a threat of being stranded in quarantine in Taiwan for two weeks. Thanks to some jumping through hoops with the help of the very accommodating Balinese and Taiwanese staff that magically rerouted our flights, we made it back to the States. It felt like I was being tested in some way to ask repeatedly: Was going home worth all this rather than staying in paradise? It was a very different world than we had left it a few weeks before. It felt like an apocalyptic dream.

In the following weeks, I questioned why I came back. There were moments of crying, yelling, anxiety, anger, and depression but they all moved through me faster than they had before. I have seen the shadows and danced with them, and now I know their steps, so I allow them to take the lead, if necessary. I shed relationships that represented instability so that I could remain as calm as possible. I made better choices in how to engage with people and the news from the outer world. The most grounding piece of all was moving home to be with Gramma and Mom as the chaos ripped through our collective lives.

What I have come to realize in these uncertain times is that nothing is certain, even what we think is certain. The only thing we can do is be present and not worry about what comes next. It's been expansive, healing, liberating, joyful, and for the most part, easeful in the surrender to change. It all stems from the awareness and the ability to make a choice in how we dance with the uncertainty of Chaos, and if

Anxiety comes, allow it to flow through: don't resist it, and ask if it might be an opportunity for expansion.

The Cocreative Chaos

We all seem to be in a state of anxiety during uncertain times. We can take a step back and observe the year 2020: the pandemic, social justice movement, elections, shootings that felt like they were becoming another daily occurrence, global warming, and so on. That is not even a look into our personal lives. We can't avoid the unknown but as I hopefully showed through my story, we have a choice in how we see it and dance with it.

What I have learned over the years is that all of it is an invitation to shift perspective. It is when we don't trust the trajectory of the chaos or it takes us in our shadows that we get lost, confused, and anxious.

As I go through my edits now and rewrite over the past few weeks, I have become even tighter with Chaos. I have even decided to reclaim it for what it truly is: the void, the gap, the liminal space, the space in between where everything created in the Universe is born from. We need Chaos to continue to deconstruct what we know to be true, to grow, and to expand as we give birth to innovations, inspirations, and creations. What needs to happen in that space is to quiet the noise we tend to call chaos. What if all the distractions and illusions of obstacles are questions to get us in the flow of co-creation itself? What if what we see as hardships are invitations into creating a new world that is trying to be birthed? What if it can't come into this reality simply because we are still holding too tightly to the old thing that needs to die?

When we get quiet, go into that space, we enter the quantum field of endless possibilities; that's where the magic happens. You must trust this magic is real and hold on for the ride! It will take you through your shadows; this adventure is not for the people who want life to just move smoothly. This is a call to adventure, of intense experience, and deep exploration of the creation that is YOU. Hold on!

Crowned in Consciousness

Another visit to the chakra system, our crown chakra, which is located at the top of our head where the crown rests for all of us queens and kings. This is where we tap into the greater consciousness. Where in those moments of chaos, there is a deep sense of trust in the Universe, or God, or whatever resonates most with you that supports you from beyond, confirming that you are being supported. It is also where anxiety is transformed from monkey-brain thinking into a more expansive experience of ourselves and remembering how we are all interconnected.

Those moments I took the biggest leaps in my life, I had to have a deep sense of trust, to take the leap and trust that the parachute would open. We might see these as synchronicities, coincidences, or signs from the Universe. While I was grieving the death of my dad, I felt his presence, sometimes so palpable. I had conversations with strangers that I swore were messages directly from him. I saw animal totems and received messages from him to pay attention to my dreams, stay where I am, or move on from a relationship. This expanded awareness is what allows us to play in the chaos. As we sit deeply into the gap of liminal space and see ourselves as a speck of dust, not as something so insignificant that we get lost, overwhelmed, or swallowed up by it but rather as an invitation to be part of the magic, to dance with it, to co-create with it! To fully realize that Chaos, that space in between heaven and earth, needs us to play our very significant role here on Earth, whether it is a speck of dust or a bright shining star, it must be played out authentically through the choices we make. Each of our souls was cast in a role, and we chose it before we got into our body. We might have forgotten the role that we chose, but the beautiful thing is the Universe reminds us through the signs to keep going or be wary. If we are paying attention, that is when Chaos works its magic; when we fight it, that is when the anxiety and overwhelm overtakes us.

Even in those scary times with my dad, I knew I was safe and that there was a deep knowing that it was all part of my role to endure. Perhaps it was to go through all that to share it with you, and to help you remember and shift your perspective. Maybe that is it, maybe it is not, maybe I will find out, maybe I will not. I am just going to keep dancing and trust it is all going to be good.

Let's Check In

Chaos can be seen and experienced as disorder and confusion. True. We can see our entire world as utterly confusing and disorienting. I can say that based on the media alone, each day is full of disorder and confusion. I ask you: How do you want to dance with it?

- Do you want to wake up every day feeling disoriented by the next wave of disorder that catapults you into a panic?

- Or do you want to feel grounded knowing that the waves will change again and again, and you get to choose how you control your life?

If it's the latter, cool. Let's get centered and grounded. Here are some ways to do that:

Centering

- Place your hands on your body and take five to ten breaths until you feel back to what feels reoriented in your body. Acknowledge your breath, how your body feels under your hands, the weight and touch of your hands on your clothes and skin. Whatever else you notice that feels real at that moment brings you back to your present moment.

- State two facts you know to be true as a mantra while you breathe, like, "My name is... I am..." I have been known to do this in a few anxious moments in my life and it always anchored me and kept me from going down the rabbit hole of disastrous thought patterns about what *could* happen.

- Or say any other soothing mantra of your choice with

five to ten breaths, like "I am safe."

Grounding

- Identify supportive surroundings that are underneath you (i.e., chair and/or floor). Connect your feet and/or hands to it for five to ten breaths. Trust it is there.

- Identify surroundings through your senses five, four, three, two, one. Observe out loud five things you see, four things you hear, three things you feel, two things you smell, one thing you taste in your present moment.

The definition of chaos through the eyes of physics addresses that we are made of chaos, the formless matter that became our Universe. Perhaps another way of seeing this is that Chaos was here long before us, so choose wisely how you play with it. There are moments it can be fun and there are moments that can feel scary, and this is where Anxiety picks up the thread.

One of my teachers, Jeanmarie Paolillo, always used to say that Anxiety and Expansion look and feel the same. I would like to take it a step further and say, they *are* the same. Anxiety simply lacks the trust that everything will be okay in the space of the unknown. When we lack Trust, Resistance, or maybe Fear, steps in.

Just like the Universe, we are always in a state of expansion from the seeds of creation.

Now, it is when we don't trust this process of expansion our friend Anxiety can show up.

In these moments Trust disappears, and Anxiety rears its ugly head, this is what I do.

I stop, breathe, listen to my body, discern, and maybe make a new choice with my friend, Curiosity.

Try it for yourself:

- **Stop.** Whatever you are doing, just put it all down for a moment.

- **Breathe.** Usually, when we forget to trust the process, we forget to flow with the energy of life (prana) and resist it, or worse, cut ourselves off from our natural flow and breath (where prana flows).

- **Listen to Your Body.** There might be a new sensation that is telling you something that wants to be acknowledged in the experience. This may come through as sensations in your body, thoughts, or emotions. Maybe it is legitimate Fear keeping you away from legitimate harm *OR* maybe it is just scared of the unknown and just needs a little TLC before you take the next step. Your body is like your own little child and wants to be heard, felt, and seen.

- **Discern.** As you listen to these sensations, thoughts, emotions that arise, have a conversation with them. Discern if Fear is necessary or if it is time to invite Curiosity into play. Ask questions, ground yourself, and see if there is a spark of joy within you that is saying, "Hey! I think it is safe! Trust this! We are ready to create, play, and expand!!"

- **Make a New Choice.** If Fear was leading you down the rabbit hole of Distrust and Anxiety, say "Thank you, but goodbye!" and send it on its way. Take Curiosity's stretched-out hand (that has been here this whole time) and ask, "What do you want to show me today so I can be the fullest expression of myself?"

Let her lead you to your ever-expanding heart space.

- **Rinse and Repeat.** When Trust (in the process) challenges you, knocks you around, or simply quiets down, rinse and repeat until you two are inseparable.

The last words of wisdom from our friends Chaos and Anxiety are that they want to be seen. So let them when the time is right. If it is you who needs to hold space for them, do it. If someone else needs to see it, show it unapologetically.

Think of both Chaos and Anxiety as little children that want attention from their mom. They start by yelling at her "looooook at me!" while swinging from a tree branch over a cliff and tugging on her clothing respectively. If Mom doesn't pay attention to the tug of baby Anxiety or even observe the little wild child Chaos swinging from the tree, they will get louder and wilder to be seen. Until it gets so out of control that Mom can't help but stop and see Anxiety's full-blown tantrum and the madness of Chaos about to leap off the tree into the abyss below.

How to observe:

- Sit with Chaos. Ask her what she wants in the space of the unknown. Is it to play and get crazy? Is it to give something that has been bottled up an expression? Is it to create something new? Is it to receive some kind of level of safety? What?

- Then, let them do it safely, whatever that means to you. Set clear boundaries for yourself if you feel that is necessary.

- If this Anxiety needs someone to see it, show it to them in a safe way. Let them know you are not trusting the situation you are in whether it is with them or that you just need another witness to let you know that you are in fact okay. Be vulnerable. You have nothing to lose, and your whole self to gain by showing all of you to someone who loves you. If they can't handle it, they judge you, or walk away from you, walk away from them. They don't deserve this wild little child that wants to be free. You will find that person or people who want to see your fullest expression. That might be the bigger lesson: to see that you will always be okay, even if just in the presence of yourself. Trust that as you step into the unknown.

Now, whatever you are feeling in this moment, finish this statement:

As I dance with Chaos and transform anxiety into expansion, my body tells the story of...

ACT THREE

GRAND JETE INTO THE SUN

First, you leap, and then you grow wings.

— *William Sloane Coffin*

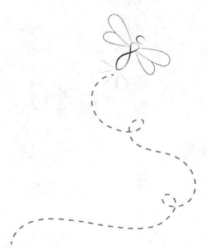

Letter to Radiant One

Hello again my Dear Radiant One,

How was it moving through the shadows? Now, we get to lean into the lightness of being. Still, some obstacles may come up and that is okay. Let whatever comes, flow through you.

My story continues as I make friends with the light and invite more dance and play into my life. I have to say through the eight years of my emotional recovery and finally feeling like I might be on the other side of it all, there are a lot more times that are filled with joy, gratitude, confidence, love, peace, trust, and inspiration. It is not as though I conquered the shadow emotions and they never returned. Please do not think this! They still come but my relationship with them has changed. For instance, when my multi-author book was released as I was writing this, Anger reared its ugly head. I had no idea it would. Sure, I was expecting Fear and Anxiety but Anger? I tapped into my resources, and it flowed through me in a matter of a day or two. It didn't linger, harbor Resentment, or harm my body as it did before and then I was able to lean into these lighter emotions like Gratitude for the opportunity to share these parts of me to help you on your path.

As we explore more of my story and the lighter emotions, remember all of it belongs. Dear Radiant One, you hold the light and the dark. We are not trying to get away from the shadows by embracing just the light. So, dive in now with this knowing.

Enjoy and celebrate all of you,

Phoebe

Letter to Gratitude and Appreciation

Dear Gratitude and Appreciation,

It took courage for me to invite you in during those darker parts of my life. I did it though.

I was taught at a very young age to send thank you letters after receiving gifts for birthdays and Christmas. I made a point not to just say a blanket statement but rather express why I was happy to receive someone's thoughtful gifts. The practice of you both was instilled in me for the better part of my life. In many ways, this book is really in honor and acknowledgment of you, Gratitude and Appreciation, through everything I have experienced: the dark, the light, the laughs, the tears, the joy, the anger, the shame, the confidence, all of it; you both have been humming underneath it this whole time.

With that said, I don't know how much I hung out with you during my teen years, as I was pretty pissed about my life circumstances of losing my childhood. I lost my home because of Dad's crack problem, left my high school to live in Texas so I would be safe, came back to live with my mom and stepdad which was a horrible transition, and left my high school again because my stepdad was going to medical school in DC. Because of all that, I was forced to go to therapy because I was labeled "the crazy one" despite keeping it relatively together through all my hardships, on top of all the other normal teenage angst, awkwardness, stress, and drama. I did try to make the best of all of it and stay positive. I can honestly say though that I do not remember feeling either of you all too often through that period of my life. I am guessing that in general, not too many teenagers connect with you during this time. Do you just lay low during those years and hope we find our way back to you later in life?

Let's be honest, my twenties weren't much better. Those were the years I was more vocal about all the hardships I had to deal with in my teens since I didn't have any sort of outlet back then. I remember many drunken brunch weekends in the city with friends, we all shared stories about whose childhood and family were worse. That was how my friends bonded back then and that was my therapy since I didn't have health insurance.

I'd like to think I spoke to the two of you when the good things happened in my life during that period: the dance opportunities, my engagement, my wedding. I hope you felt me observing you during those moments. If you did not, I am truly sorry, Gratitude and Appreciation.

I remember how my focus intentionally shifted to you both when I was thirty. One of my teachers, Jillian Pranksy, sent out a monthly newsletter and she shared about her practice of Gratitude for forty days to shift her perspective. I was intrigued by this practice, so I decided to give it a try. I started to write in my journal every day as my practice. Things began to shift and despite my busy and stressful city life, my heart felt a bit lighter, and I didn't feel as stressed. Social media wasn't a thing yet, so I began sending emails to my friends, family, and students to encourage them to practice too. I sent each day my reflections and prompted them to reflect upon you Gratitude, in their own ways. We kept doing this for a couple of years and I found when I needed you most was during the holidays when I felt more stressed than usual. With all the Christmas shopping, the baking and cooking, the holiday parties, the colder weather, and the traveling, I strived to make everything special yet ended up feeling anxious and began to loathe it all. I set the intention to shift my perspective and led "40 days of Gratitude" from Thanksgiving to New Year each year.

As I reflect on it all now, I can see how you both called on me in preparation for those darker days that were just upon me then.

In 2012, I ran a forty-day practice on social media with my students at the yoga program I was directing. I remember the posts included Gratitude for my husband, my dad, my new dream home, my dog, my new yoga program, which turned out to be all things that would no longer be in my life by the time I circled to the next year's annual practice. Eight days after that forty-day practice in 2012 concluded with my students, my dad was found dead. How could I feel you two then, Gratitude and Appreciation? How could that have even been possible?

But somehow, I found you. I found you in my mom's arms when she got in her car and drove to me that day. I saw and heard you in the laughs and tears of his best friends at his AA club where we held his funeral. I felt you close that morning in March when I finally woke up without pain in my heart and knew everything was going to be okay. Even though a few hours later I would find out my marriage was ending, I knew you were with me, holding my hand saying, "And this too, is going to be a gift. Just hold on, Phoebe."

Through the process of detangling myself from a man I had been with for fifteen years, I felt you both in the night he told me he would set me free and signed our divorce papers because he knew I could not go on the dark path he was choosing for himself. My heart broke for the path he was choosing, but I was silently grateful it was no longer mine to walk.

I found you when I had my breakthrough and didn't go to work and instead drove to my mom's and she told me to follow my heart. I felt you when I was graced with Dad's estate money that allowed me to go to Costa Rica where I began to envision a new life.

There were so many magical encounters during that year with "strangers" that I know both of you had a hand in. I know this because the more I called out to you both, Gratitude and Appreciation, the more magical opportunities unfolded for me from the subtle to the extraordinary.

You both have been close, these last eight years especially, and I promise to continue to acknowledge you for the rest of my journey. I am not sure how I would have survived without you if it wasn't for the two of you holding my hand during those darker days and showing me there was a reason for all of it. You kept telling me to keep going forward but to look back once in a while to see the beautiful tapestry we were weaving together. This makes looking forward a whole lot more exciting, imagining the mystery of what could be next for us.

Thank you so much.

With deep love and acknowledgment,

Phoebe

Gratitude as a Gateway Drug

You can think of Gratitude and Appreciation as the gateway drug to all our lighter emotions. If we are grateful, we can transform our darker emotions like Anger, Resentment, Fear, Guilt, and Anxiety into Joy, Happiness, Peace, Serenity, and Enthusiasm. We also begin to trust ourselves and the choices we make because we realize that even within the difficult choices we made/make, there are lessons and gifts we did not originally foresee. This also builds more Confidence in taking leaps forward. When we are in the flow with Gratitude and Appreciation, Inspiration also flows effortlessly.

During my time in Bali, I fell in love with how devotional the people are there. They share offerings to their gods in so many ways, one being at mealtime. They offer a little bit of their food on the side of their dish to the gods as a thank you. I believe this is one of the reasons Balinese smile more than us Westerners. Try it some time. Give up a little something you might not need with gratitude to something/someone else and see how it feels. Perhaps you will appreciate what you *do* a little bit more and enjoy being generous more often.

A Grateful Heart

When I sat with the lighter emotions and how I wanted to organize them to align with the chakras, I paused for a bit since I felt that these emotions dance throughout the chakra system. Love and Connection seem to be the no-brainer to align with the heart chakra, but as I said before, Gratitude is the gateway to all the lighter emotions and because of that, it must begin at the center of our heart and radiate outward from there.

When we express gratitude for someone, at least in Eastern cultures, we bring our hands to the heart and bow in acknowledgment. When we say grace at the dinner table, we may do the same here as well. This is where Gratitude begins, in the heart.

On our most wretched days and periods of our life, we may come to a gratitude practice to find a way to possibly change our connection with ourselves and the world. Don't just think of it as rewiring to change the patterns of the mind but to tap us back into our heart space, to move us to the rhythm of our heartbeat and breath again.

When gratitude and appreciation of our world become the focal point in our heart, the other little annoyances of our lives seem to take less hold and make space for more Love, Connection, Joy, Peace.

Think about it for a moment. When you are having a bad day and someone says, "Just be happy!" or "Just relax!" or "Trust someone out there loves you!" Depending on how wretched you feel, you might just want to tell them to shove it up somewhere else that is not in their heart space. But if someone says, "This day feels like a bad one, but is there something you can still be grateful for?" You probably can find something, even if it is just the smell of your new shampoo. Gratitude can be that subtle but can make quite a big wave of change quickly when practiced earnestly.

Gratitude can be the disruptor when we are on the hamster wheel of dark emotions. In Buddhism, there is a word, *shenpa,* that means "hook" or these days we might even say "triggered." When I was married, I read a lot of Pema Chödrön books, and I even turned John on to reading a couple. When we both noticed the other one got hooked or triggered by our day's events and were spiraling into an old thought pattern, we would acknowledge it and say what we were grateful for at that moment. It allowed both of us a space to pause from the downward spiral of the old way of thinking and tap back into the present experience of life. I will say, it is important to acknowledge at the first notice of the hook, rather than in a full-blown downward spiral, but it can still make a difference if you are committed to the practice.

Let's Check In

Gratitude Journal. You probably know about this and there seem to be dozens of journals out there you can buy. Here are a couple of ways I inspired my groups in the past for our 40 Days of Attitude of Gratitude Challenge:

- **Simple version.** List three things you are grateful for about each day.

- **Past/Present/Future.** Write down a challenging lesson from your past, why you are grateful for it in your present (or something else), and why you can see you may be grateful for it in your future.

- **Person, Place, Thing.** Each day write a person, place, thing you are grateful for.

- **Inspiring Quote.** If you enjoy quotes like I do, go through a poetry book or a book you are reading each morning, and choose a line to reflect upon. See how you can experience it throughout your day. Write at the end of the day how you are grateful for that new perspective.

- **Flip the Switch.** Let yourself vent about all the crappy things in your life and then on the next page, follow up with how each of those things may also bring gratitude.

Appreciation of what you have.

- **The Little Things.** Every time you have a meal or receive a gift throughout your day, say a little prayer or thanks for how it came to you, who made it, where it came from.

- **Call a Friend.** Call, text, email, or even snail mail a different friend once a week and share with them why you appreciate them being in your world (you can also do this to initiate making new friends).

- **Spread the Gratitude**. If you enjoy social media, share your practice with others there and inspire them to join you.

- **Whenever You Can Say Thanks, Do It.** Acknowledge the small gestures made by friends, acquaintances, strangers, and especially yourself whenever you can.

- **Fall in Love with Nature.** Go somewhere in nature that you love: the mountains, the beach, the quiet spot in your yard. Wherever you feel the most comfortable, safe, or connected, and dive into your surroundings. Meditate, dance, write in a journal, and most importantly observe what is all around you and is loving you back. Listen to the birdsongs, see the little insects or animals that come to visit, talk with them, and ask them questions, feel the grass between your toes, or the cool water from another river on your body. Be in your surroundings and communion with nature.

Now, whatever you are feeling in this moment, finish this statement:

With Gratitude and Appreciation, I embody the story of...

Letter to Trust and Patience

Dear Trust and Patience,

There are so many ways to look at the two of you. Where shall I start? My relationship with you is a rather complicated one. Let's start with you, Trust. I feel like we were pretty tight for a while when I was very young. You were my link to Intuition. As a child, I was extremely intuitive, which was a blessing for a little bit because you kept me safe, but then I felt we got our signals crossed and it felt more like a curse.

When I was very young, I trusted the people I was supposed to trust: my parents, my mom's side of the family being Grandpop Bob, Gramma, and my aunts. I did not feel good around my dad's parents or his brother. I always got bad feelings being around them. There were several times I got car sick going to see them. I felt it in my gut and could not stomach having to be around them when they said awful things to me about how I wasn't perfect like my older half-sister who got straight A's, won swimming meets, and did whatever it was that I wasn't doing. I also hated that I could not bring my friends or even talk about my friends simply because they were a different color than me or from a different country. I also felt the stress of my mom and my dad who had to white-knuckle their way through conversations with my grandparents. I often wondered why we had to go at all.

I trusted warm people and could immediately trust myself to feel when to steer away from the colder people, particularly grownups. I felt when it was safe to go on adventures with my friends in our neighborhood's parks or just beyond the parameters into hidden trails.

Things got complicated though when the people I felt were warm and could trust, like my mom and dad, began to deceive me. The night that they split up, my contract with you Trust, felt null and void. I was still grateful for you in the moments you and Intuition kept me safe during Dad's episodes, but our relationship shifted. I felt moments before when he went into his flashbacks or flipped the switch to rage. Trust, you were there leading me to Intuition to get out of the way and take cover. However, the messages you sent me are what made me feel cursed. Your voice was so strong and powerful that I began to think I was creating these moments. So, after a while, I turned your voice down and stopped listening to you. You were still there though, which now I am grateful for. You kept me safe in so many ways and gave me amazing opportunities along the journey.

The opportunities are what I want to celebrate now. That year it was time to apply to college and I started to plan for my dream path as a dancer. I knew

I was applying to colleges that my family could not afford (my mom could not even afford for me to go to a community college if I wanted to). I auditioned for all the dance programs anyway and applied for all the scholarships, grants, and loans, I could find. I received some but still not enough for my mom to handle the rest. Since my dad was off being a drug addict and possibly homeless, there was no more counting on him.

It was coming closer to the time to send in my acceptance and my first payment to my first-choice school, the University of the Arts. My older half-sister was graduating from college-fully funded by my grandparents' trust fund for her—something they never thought to set up for me because they thought so little of me and felt it was my dad's responsibility to take care of me.

My mom told me I had to go accompany them to West Virginia for my half-sister's graduation and ask them for money to attend college. I loathed that this is what I was going to have to do after all the years that they made me feel so worthless. I had zero desire to beg them for money and make me feel even smaller than they made me feel before. Trust, you whispered in my ear to go and to not ask them for anything, to just sit with Patience and wait. So, I did just that. I went and waited for it. I waited through the very long car ride while my grandparents bickered the entire way there. I suffered through an entire night in a sorority house with drunk people, and even though I didn't drink at that time, I felt intoxicated. I had to share a bunk bed with my half-sister's boyfriend's brother who tried to take advantage of me, and I heard you say, "Just wait, don't make waves, it will get better." I remember at some point finding my half-sister in the bathroom, drunk and crying about how she felt so bad that I had to deal with Dad alone. I was a bit resentful that I had to be so strong to let her know I was fine and was going to be fine, when no one ever told me that I was actually going to be fine, except you, Trust and Patience. When it felt like all the people in my world were betraying me by ignoring the big fat elephant in the room that Dad was not a dad at all, and that I had to somehow fend for myself because no one looked out for me, you two told me I would be okay and to just hold on. You told me I was going to get out of this mess and be able to be free and be with people soon who would get me.

At some point, during the weekend I saw my grandpa go off with my half-sister to have what looked to be a serious conversation. I knew it was about my money. I didn't know what, how, or why but Trust, you told me it was coming soon, very soon, and I wasn't going to have to beg these people. I remember calling my mom from the payphone at the graduation right after Mr. Rogers came out for the keynote speech and sang "It's a Beautiful Day in the Neighborhood." The same Mr. Rogers who was friends with my Grandpop Bob who had died just a few months before. For some strange reason, I felt my Grandpop Bob was sending me a message. He was telling me that it was going to be a beautiful day, that I could go to whatever college I wanted and be the biggest fish in the biggest pond that I wanted to be in. He was telling me that these neighbors—my grandparents—were finally going to make it right in my world.

My mom asked with great anticipation on the other line, "Did you ask your grandparents for the money?" I replied, "No, but it is going to be fine."

Trust and Patience, you truly tested me that day! It wasn't until the very last moment of that weekend when my mom came to pick me up in a clown car packed with other relatives visiting. My grandpa pulled Mom and me aside and said to come to sit in his study. Nana probably stayed outside to make sure no one stole or broke any of her precious antiques. He sat us down and said he was going to pay for my college from my sister's trust fund (which also later bought her a Range Rover, grad/Ph.D. schools, and other gifts, after they were done paying for my school). They sent me the very minimal amount to survive after my grants, scholarships, and loans covered what was needed. It was the only time in my life they did anything generous for me, and it wasn't any extra skin off their backs since it was already set aside for her. I didn't care how or why though; I was just so grateful for the two of you who told me to hold on.

Trust, you were there other times too that felt like magic. The time I was accepted to go to the summer dance festival, Jacob's Pillow. Again, I knew at the audition that I would be accepted but didn't have the funds. I magically received a gift from John's dad, who ended up being my father-in-law further down the line, but at that point, he had only met me maybe once or twice before. And the time I was accepted to the program to dance in Italy and again did not have the money. I saw myself there and sure enough, I got there with a little inheritance my mom received the month before. She gave it to me so I could make my dream of dance and travel a reality.

All those moments in my life I was a stereotypical poor starving artist living in New York City. I had started to rack up some credit card debt because waiting tables and dancing were not covering rent and bills. You both told me it would be okay, to just hold on that the money would come. At twenty-five, I had $10k in credit card debt and student loans, yet I fully believed in the message you sent me to keep with the Pilates training. Within two months of getting my certification, leaving my waitressing gig, I started booking clients out of what felt like nowhere, making three times what I was making at the restaurant easily. I was able to pay off my debt within six months. Done.

From that, we were tight again but when John started abusing drugs, my relationship wavered with him and you, Trust. I was always looking for clues or evidence that he was hiding something from me, consciously and unconsciously. I questioned him and I questioned myself. Our shaky relationship of the past was triggered, and I was again unsure if I was somehow playing a hand in creating it, so I turned the other way and tried not to look.

Before these times, Patience, we were pretty good. Aside from the Christmas present excitement when I would sneak in all the ways to find out what I was getting from Santa, I was a pretty laid-back person and allowed the timing of life to unfold as it was intended to be. But when Trust and I wavered around John, I became weary of you too, Patience. If I am being really honest, I think it began the year of my marriage. I thought perhaps his partying would calm down a bit, but it didn't. He traveled more for work, and when he came back from tours, he shared these wild stories of working insane hours on projects and almost not getting the music done in time for the concert. Then would come back home to spend a week (or two) on what he called a "bender" of getting super drunk and high as his way of decompressing, followed by getting deathly sick. I had to wake him up on the couch early one morning as I left to go teach and realized he had thrown up on our couch in his sleep. I wanted things to change but I grew less trusting and less patient that they would.

I started to force situations to happen, like getting a cat, then moving so we could keep the cat, then wanting a dog, then wanting to move out of the city, then wanting to buy a house. All these things I wanted because you both, Trust and Patience, were not present, and I was flailing. I felt like I was being thrown around in a snow globe in my marriage and didn't know which direction was up or down and whatever direction I would head, didn't feel right. I did whatever I could but the two of you felt quieter and quieter the more I searched for you.

There was a time in the midst of the flailing that I saw a glimpse of you again: the day Dad called me after his eighteen-year disappearance. When I heard his voice, I knew. I heard you both in his voice telling me it was safe, and it was worth the wait. I felt calm, peace, joy, happiness, love, and connection flood my body. My daddy was alive, healthy, sober, and safe. He helped me see my North Star for a bit during those four years we reconnected.

For the last eight years, Trust and Patience, we have been rebuilding our relationship again. There have been times when I veered away from you both, like when I fell in love with my very dear friend, San Diego. I just don't think we were on solid ground yet and whatever he said or did once we entered into a romantic relationship, I could not believe he was real or telling me the truth. Trust and Patience, I ended up testing him and pushing him away so many times over our three years of the on and off relationship. Then, I just lost him. Like that, it was all gone. I think he just got so fed up with my lack of faith in you two that he just went off and had a baby with someone else.

That was a huge wake-up call to get my relationship tight with you both again or my whole life would be lived in paranoia. Since then, I feel we are stronger than ever. Patience, when I get a little bit anxious, you whisper to me that it will all be okay, that I will be able to receive love like that again, an even bigger love that I will never have to question. Trust, you come over and wrap your warm arms around me and I can feel your steadiness, so I relax completely.

I don't know what my future will look like, but it feels good knowing I have you both on my side again. I feel you both in my bones, so there is no more wavering. I stand with my two feet planted and you two beside me, holding a solid ground for me.

Our story continues to unfold slowly, gracefully, at the pace it is intended to be. I know your voices better than I know my own now, or maybe you are my voice now. Thank you for not giving up on me.

With grace,

Phoebe

Choices Based in Trust

Trust is our foundation where we feel safe, stable, secure. If we don't feel safe with the people who love us, the situations, and places we are in, then how can we trust anything, including ourselves? Some of us take this for granted, others who have endured trauma in their life lose a sense of trust, feel betrayed, and perhaps even feel lost in finding it again. I think we have all experienced this at some level at some point in our lives.

If there is little to no trust, then how can we be patient about anything? Patience is intimately linked with Trust. If we trust everything is working out in our favor—even the hard moments—then it is impossible to feel impatient. Now we are not talking about when we might get excited and a little impatient because Enthusiasm is present. Even then there is a deep sense of trust. We are talking about the impatience that is accompanied by anxiety, for example: *if this doesn't happen now my whole life is going to crumble.* Do you know what I mean? The desperation, as if your whole life is a Jenga game and if you don't move that one piece at the right moment the whole thing will collapse, and you feel like that moment must be NOW!

So, when you are in these kinds of states of being, how do you cope? When you don't feel like you can trust the person you are with, the situation you are in, the toxic work environment, or the unhealthy choices you are making, what do you do to feel safe again?

What do you do when you feel Distrust's naughty little friend Impatience in your ear saying, "Why isn't it happening now?" or "Why *is* this happening now?" or "This can't happen now!" or "My whole life is going to fall apart if this doesn't happen now!" What do you do?

Rooted in Trust

As you may have already guessed, Trust and Patience reside and feel balanced in the root chakra because it is so intimately connected with Fear. When our basic needs are met and we don't fear our future, we can trust our needs will be met.

Trust is the bedrock for everything. If trust lacks a solid foundation, everything above it crumbles. This goes for our physical and subtle bodies as well. If we don't feel we can trust our support, we don't feel like we have a solid leg to stand on, physically and metaphorically. It is important to feel we can trust our bodies and the choices it makes to keep us safe. Just as we looked at with Fear, Trust is linked to keeping us safe with fight, flight, or freeze (the sympathetic nervous system) responses. We must trust the body will run when we are in danger, fight when we need to stand up for ourselves to keep us safe, and know when to just pause. Trust is also what allows us to rest and digest (parasympathetic nervous system) when we get the message that it is safe to do so.

The moment I felt I could trust myself is when I felt the safest and had nothing to fear. When Fear was not present, I trusted even more deeply. There is a part of me that has a fear of sharing so much in these pages with you, yet I completely trust it is necessary and I can relax into that knowing. My body feels safe, my hand is steady as I write this, and I know in my bones it is meant to be. I often say that phrase too when it comes to trust, "I know it in my bones." I am not sure what chakra that would be categorized as but I feel bones are also foundational, at the root of our body. Our bones give us structure, the form for everything else in our body to take shape. Trust is our bedrock for everything to build and take shape on.

Let's Check In

This is a really big one. First things first, you must ground your body and feel safe in it again. If you don't feel safe and trust your own body, then how can you move with any sort of trust in your life?

These are a few simple grounding practices that can help you get there:

Centering in Your Body. Simply place your hands on your body (hands-on heart and/or belly) and take five to ten slow, deep, calming, and cleansing breaths.

I like to use mantra when I feel out of alignment with how I feel. This year's mantra for me has simply been Trust. Whenever you feel impatient or not quite sure if things are moving in a direction that feels safe, simply close your eyes, breathe, and say to yourself "Trust" for five to ten breaths and see how you feel. You might just need that simple re-centering to trust again, or you may feel that something is off and there is a new choice to make to realign you.

Centering in Your Being. When you need to build trust in your present experience you can say a simple mantra that anchors you in the present moment such as "My name is... I am..." and say a fact that you know to be absolutely true like your age or what color shirt you are wearing.

Grounding. Whatever you do, focus on the first chakra to feel grounded, rooted, and safe again. This can be yoga, restorative or yin yoga, meditation, tai chi, yardwork, eating root vegetables, whatever you need to do to trust and feel safe within your body and your surroundings. It is not a one-size-fits-all, do things you know feel good and anchor you back into your body, your surroundings, and your present experience. The more you do this, the more of what you do not trust will come into focus, and you can see more clearly what it is to make new choices to align with what you want and can trust.

Create a Safe Place. If being in your present experience does not feel safe, you can also imagine a Safe Place where you feel you can relax without the threat of stress/danger. Use an image of your past, or if you don't have a direct experience, imagine a scenario where you felt safe and could trust what was around you. What would that support feel like in your body to receive it now? The more your body can feel the safety and relax into it, the more you can see with a clearer perspective.

If you have the freedom to physically create that safe place in your own home, do it. The more you can feel relaxed at home (and in your body) the more you can trust life. Clear out anything that carries the weight of your past or tells you a story of not making the right choices for your present or future. When you feel supported by your surroundings, you can relax into the possibilities that flow to you and through you effortlessly, with Patience and Trust.

Now, whatever you are feeling in this moment, finish this statement:

As I step into my life with more Trust and Patience, I embody the story of...

Letter to Enthusiasm and Inspiration

Dear Enthusiasm and Inspiration,

When you two come over to play, there is a divine flow of you both. I always convince myself it will last forever but it never does. It feels like you two are fairies that pop into my view for no one else to see. Sometimes that can be fun like it's our little secret, but other times it is unbelievably frustrating because I want other people to see you, feel you, hear you, and they just don't! When I tell them about the ideas you share with me, they just look right through me as if I am not there or with perplexity like I somehow randomly grew another head while I was speaking to them.

Dance has always been my connection with you both. If I felt any sort of disconnection, music and movement were a direct path to you and you both were immediately ready to play anytime and anywhere.

Ever since I was a child, I could play a song and feel Inspiration's presence. Sometimes you simply wanted me to move my body around through space, but other times you held my attention in stillness as you showed me a whole dance to choreograph including all the shapes, formations of people, the colors, and all the energy needed to bring it to life from one transition to the other. Sometimes, if I was really lucky, you would show me a whole dance of my life. You would part the curtains to show me the flow of people in and out of it entering and exiting stage right and left, the high moments as lifts, and the lower ones as falls or rolls to ground to recover with grace, the bright lights and upbeat music of celebratory moments, the dark corners where I cried alone, the slow and sensual duets, the energized upbeat groups moving in union. I could see how I was to play my role in it all.

Then Inspiration, you would pass me off to Enthusiasm for her to do her work on me. Enthusiasm, you seemed to always run at high speed and burn a bright vibrant light on both ends. It was hard to sustain that for myself when I didn't have the energy of others to play off. When I lacked the resources to get others onboard your fun train, I felt so blinded by the disorientating combination of your light and their dimwittedness, that I stumbled around bumping into things as I jumped up and down full of you in their dark and vacant rooms. That's when I decided to quiet you down a bit, by trying to contain you so I wasn't judged by others. When your energy was no longer sustainable, I would become so depleted of my own energy that I would just crash, especially after a dance performance.

Experiencing the highs and lows of you both made me weary for a while because your energy had such extremes. Having a father with bipolar made my relationship with you complicated. When I felt your high energy run through me and didn't want it to end, I would begin to wonder if I was having a manic episode and if my fate would soon lead me to crash and burn. But I love you both and am very grateful for our closeness since I see how so many people barely know who you are or choose not to connect with you for their reasons of not having enough time, too many obligations, or not feeling worthy of you.

In the last several years, I have learned how to harness you a bit better, so your energy flows to me and through me more easefully and sustainably. I started to connect with you differently through nature. I often put my feet in the grass, sand, or water to ground me in your flow. I observe the vibrant colored butterflies fluttering from flower to flower, the deer and baby foxes frolicking with their mamas, the birds chirping their sweet songs just bursting with the two of you, Inspiration and Enthusiasm. It all makes me feel more connected with your natural flow and I trust it is endless.

As I write this, it makes me think of humans locked in the screens (myself included as I type this), how they stress about if the numbers in their bank will pay for their kid's camp, groceries, or rent, or people who claim to be too busy to have fun. How did we get so locked up in our heads and our screens? How did we get further away from the flow of living connected, integrated lives with you two, Enthusiasm and Inspiration?

I remember when I lived in New York City, I took long walks through Central Park and Riverside instead of the train after seeing a client or taking a class. I got lost in those spaces with you both, and I felt your flow take over me. I felt so light and free in my body, mind, and heart. As I left the tree-lined streets moving back into the urban concrete jungle, you hummed with me until I got home and entered my apartment. Then I would be back into reality. John quickly jerked me back in with the bombardment of work drama he was dealing with, or what the dog or co-worker did to piss him off. There was usually a murder mystery ominously playing in the background and weighing down any residual light I still had of the two of you. My lightness of being with the two of you immediately dissolved into the ether and I unconsciously watched a wet blanket cover up the flow of your energy. It took me a few years to realize this. I felt a bit guilty and confused when I realized how much more energy I had with the two of you when I moved out of my marriage.

Since being single and having agency over my environment (to a certain extent), you two come over to play at a moment's notice again. It feels so good to be with you like that again, Inspiration and Enthusiasm. My promise to the three of us is that I will keep our connection lines open and allow more possibilities of connection to grow, like how I am writing with you now, or attracting more like-minded friends who enjoy cocreating with me, or anything else you point me in the direction of. I am open to your possibilities because I know you both can be anywhere and everywhere. The closer we become and the more time we spend together, the more I want everything to be infused with you both. Life is too short not to have you in it. Thank you for always giving me these gifts to enjoy alone and to share with others that are also open to your divine flow.

We need more of you and my hope is our ever-expanding universe will never run out of either of you, as you are the fuel that keeps us going!

With a very energetic hug,

Phoebe

The Secret to Enthusiasm

It is such a gift to have a zest for life. I feel blessed to have been able to tap into that throughout most of my life, but I know so many people have only touched it or maybe felt a gentle hint of a breeze of it. One of my missions in life is to change this. We need more people in our world who are open to inspiration for creation and are enthusiastic about the possibilities of what life can be. What is essential to tap into inspiration for creativity is to take away the noise, the outer chatter of what others think you should be doing, the media, the societal constraints, and whatever else you feel pulls you away from your center.

The secret is when you tap into this space, you don't always want to come back into the real world or rather you want to bring more of your inspirational world back into this reality; we need that!

Think about a child who is ready to do anything they dream of; think of the glee on their faces. What if you could have that every day of your adult life in some way? What if you could be in awe of what you get to do and be, each and every day? I believe it is possible and I want that so badly for you.

An Inspired Sacral Flow

The sacral chakra is where creation and pleasure are born. You can think of the mother's womb creating a healthy ecosystem for her baby to grow, or a home for all the ingredients to mix together and create all the possibilities for the baby to play out when it's her time to grow and expand.

This is where our creative energy flows like a river. The element associated with this chakra is water. When we are stuck or stagnant in our creative flow or when our wires are not connecting with Inspiration or Enthusiasm, our energy looks like a backed-up stream with sticks and leaves or a stagnant pool of unhealthy water. When I speak to creativity and inspiration, I am not speaking to just the artists out there. We all are creative beings. Our souls choose our bodies, our parents, our life circumstances to play out new stories, which is an act of creation. When I began believing this way, it helped me make sense of the challenges I faced over my lifetime. It has kept me from thinking like a victim in how things are happening *to* me and instead I see myself as a cocreator in how things are happening *with* me.

Think about it for a second, whatever you might be going through in your life right now. Ask the following: What is challenging? Why is this happening right now? What can I learn from it? How can I create a new option out of it?

Making new choices for our lives is a creative act. What helps us get there are our dear friends, Inspiration and Enthusiasm. We must be inspired enough to see outside of the options that are right there in front of us, even if it is the smallest new choice that we make, it can lead us to seeing an exhilarating new perspective which leads to opening to more options, more new choices, and so on. All of this is what helps us get into what some call a "flow state" of being—when everything seems to flow effortlessly for us, carrying us away from being the victim of life happening *to us*, to transforming us into seeing the bigger picture of how everything is connected and happening *with us* and *for us.*

When I contemplated which chakra this chapter would align with, I was slightly challenged for a moment. Inspiration is usually referred to as something outside of ourselves. The root word means "to be breathed" as if a divine or supernatural being brings into ourselves a new idea. This would be more aligned with the crown chakra which I do not disagree with. However, as I dive more deeply into my relationship with Chaos, I am coming to believe more that creativity is born in the depths of our being, in a dark space, a gap, a void, a place where all matter comes together to create a universe. In numerous visualizations, I have seen my womb creating life over lifetimes. But just like any literal birth, there is a breath of new life from something beyond the womb space, the father enters the space to cocreate this life. He "breathes into" the space for a great possibility for something new to be born. This all happens within the sacral space of a woman, and it translates into all our energetic bodies. This is where our polarities of energies, masculine and feminine, come together to inspire something new to be born with great enthusiasm and a deep belief that all can come to be. Whether you identify as a woman or not, the sacral space is infused with Inspiration and Enthusiasm so our lives can thrive creatively.

Let's Check In

Take a bit of time and sit with a journal with these questions. Another idea is to record these questions and play them back to yourself when you are in a quiet space, maybe on a walk in nature.

- Where are you on the enthusiasm scale about your life right now?

- Do you look forward to waking up each day or dread the alarm clock?

- Do you have a long list of "I should" or "I need to" or do you have a long list of "I get to" and "I want to"?

- What inspires you?

- Who inspires you?

- What do you create or nurture in your life that you are excited about and love to share with others?

- What do you want to create in your life but have a block around? What obstacles are getting in the way that keep you from Inspiration and Enthusiasm?

- If you are not sure about what you want to create, what are you curious about?

Once you have an idea of where you are on the spectrum of Enthusiasm and Inspiration, you can tap into the flow of them more easily at any time. It all comes down to doing what you love first and adding in a fresh perspective.

Turn Off the News. This also means turning off or removing yourself from anything else that distracts you (including your phone), that keeps you from feeling good about yourself and doing what you love, guilt and shame-free. Allow yourself to be in the darkness, the bleakness, the silence, for Inspiration to speak to you.

Walk in Nature. Explore somewhere new or set an intention to see it differently. Interact with it in a new way. If you tend to walk fast, slow down. If you tend to sit and meditate by the water, dance, and play in the stream. If you live in a city, go for a walk in a neighborhood you have not explored before. Be a tourist in your backyard!

Listen and Dance to Music that is different from your normal playlist and see if there is something new for you to be enthusiastic about.

Watch or Read a Different Genre you do not normally pick (but are still somewhat interested in).

Go to a Museum, See a Play, or do something outside of your normal box and see how your brain fires up in a new way.

Try the Normal Things in a New Way. Brush your teeth or write a note with your non-dominant hand. Laugh at yourself when it gets a little sloppy and just see if there is something new in that experience for you.

Now, whatever you are feeling in this moment, finish this statement:

As I surrender into the flow of Enthusiasm & Inspiration, I embody the story of...

Letter to Confidence and Strength

Dear Confidence and Strength,

I found you both most often through dance, my training ground.

Confidence, we met at a very young age when I knew dance was my gift and I had no doubt I would be a star—you told me that. As a child, it all came somewhat easy to me, no one ever questioned my gift or ability. Dad would give me pep talks during my post-dinner dance performances about how I could be and do anything I wanted. I might not have gotten the leading roles right away, but I was always just grateful to be doing what I loved and was good at. Then the acknowledgments came. I made co-captain of poms, got the lead role as Sandy in Grease, danced in a pre-professional dance company in middle school where I got to train with professional dancers, and was invited to be a part of professional projects from time to time. It flowed pretty easily for me there for a while.

Then around my sophomore year of high school, I started to face some challenges. That's when Strength, you came in to help me. I was trying to figure out the best route to take for my gift. I was suddenly being phased out from the dance company for no apparent reason. The director/choreographer was cold to me and started to play favorites when choosing roles. I still had my duets and solos, but it was clear I was not a favorite when she criticized me in front of the other dancers or worse, blatantly treated me as if I wasn't even there. It was heartbreaking because that company felt like home to me for years when my real home was extremely unsteady and transitional. Within that year, I moved out of my dad's house to live with my gramma in Houston for a semester, and then back to Maryland to live with my mom and stepdad. The only thing that felt steady was my rehearsal schedule, but I also knew there was something bigger out there for me.

That's when I got another opportunity to be a featured role in a dinner theater gig. It all came to a head when I had to choose between the two: my dance company which I was loyal to or a new opportunity. The callbacks for the featured role and my dance performance were all on the same day, so I decided to somehow make magic happen and do both. My family was there for my performance, including my Grandpop Bob who drove five hours from Pittsburgh.

The day went like this: I had the audition in the morning and still could potentially drive thirty minutes to get to tech rehearsal and the performance. But the audition went longer than I expected, and I had to return for the callback later that day. As I sat with my boyfriend outside the college where the auditions were being held, we planned out the whole scenario and how it could all work out. Mind you, there were no cell phones to call anyone to let them know our plan. He rushed me to my show. I missed tech and the director was so pissed at me that she cut me from the entire show except for the big number at the end; she cut me from my duets and solos that my family came to see me perform. I was embarrassed and devastated. To top it off, the show was running late, and it looked like if I stayed for the show, I wouldn't make it back in time for the callbacks. I was conflicted and Confidence, we wavered.

Then a miracle happened. As I sat backstage watching my dance performed by my understudy, my mom came backstage with a message from my Grandpop Bob that said to leave and go to that audition. Grandpop Bob was a musician, who sincerely knew what it was like to live the artist's life and paved the way for me to live it confidently. He took one look at the quality of the other dancers and said that it was time for me to leap to something bigger and better. Strength, you stood me up, walked me out knowing I could never go back to that dance company. I got myself back to the callback in time and got the gig. Grandpop Bob came back to see his granddaughter play Princess of Ababu later that summer.

That day and that experience changed my life. I believed in both of you, Strength and Confidence, and trusted the Universe was supporting me.

Confidence, a couple of years later you whispered to me to go for an open call to Dreamgirls at my new high school. It was a predominantly Black show, and I didn't know anyone yet. It was my junior year and we moved again. At that point, I resigned to be the quiet new girl and didn't make much effort to make friends since I only had two more years of high school and was tired of all the moving around I had been doing the last few years. No one knew me and they didn't know that this white girl could dance. I was nervous for various reasons, including still being scarred by my last dance company, so I stood in the back.

About five counts of eight into the combination, the choreographer stopped everything and said, "Girl, what is your name?" I looked around until I realized she was talking in my direction, "You are fierce!" Everyone looked back at me, and I looked beyond myself with no one behind me, I am sure I was beet red. I said in a very shy voice, "Me?" She pulled me downstage to the front of the group to demonstrate the sequence. I hesitated for a minute feeling distrust. I worried that the music would come on and I would dance, and everyone would laugh at me, the white girl trying to dance in Dreamgirls. But then, Confidence, you got in my ear and whispered, "Just dance, girl. You were born for this." So, I did, and I rocked it. The choreographer even made a special dance role and solos for me. I made a whole new group of friends which made my new high school life a whole lot more enjoyable.

It felt good again to be a part of a community of friends who accepted me, and I was grateful for the other opportunities I had outside of that show when it was over. Our choreographer, Shawn, was such a bright light for us. She knew how to build us up, test our strength, will, and passion, and push us to our greatest potential to get us to confidently and unapologetically shine like the stars we were. I will forever be grateful for Shawn leading me back to you both, Confidence and Strength.

When I went to college, I was tested again. It took me a little while to find you both in Philadelphia over all the noise of the many teachers and students that all seemed to have their neuroses that were projected onto me in some way. I made it through though and moved on up to New York City!

There the noise got louder, but I managed to keep you both pretty close even among hundreds of other dancers in tiny, cramped rooms for auditions.

As a child, I watched Dick Clark's New Year's Rockin' Eve every year and saw the thousands of people celebrating the new year in Times Square. I wished every year when I watched on my tiny TV screen, that I would make it there someday, and one day, I did. My first big audition after moving to the city was for

David Parsons's New Year's Eve/Times Square project in 1999. Not only did I make it to Times Square on my first NYE in New York, but I got to perform there, on the new millennium, the moment of truth for Y2K. I was dancing (and getting paid!) about a couple of hundred feet away from the ball dropping, with VIP treatment, with my warm cot and catering above Tower Records. I didn't have to stand outside in the cold with drunk idiots (part of the dream I did not envision as a child). Confidence, I rode your wave high that time.

The following eleven years in the city ebbed and flowed with you, as it should as life tested me with numerous cattle-call auditions, few callbacks, and endless late-night rehearsals for little or no pay. So many moments I woke up and questioned, what is this all for? Was it for my ego? Did anyone even care about the work or my gift as they barely looked at my headshot or my dancing and said, "Thank you, next!" So much doubt flowed between us and got in our way.

But there were moments, Strength and Confidence, we all just knew. Like the time I showed up to an all-day audition. There were over two hundred other girls there for one company role. I walked in, put my dance bag on the floor, and I just knew I was going to get it. Each combination, every cut, down to the very last one with two other dancers, I knew it was mine. We each had to travel through space with our partner, take a huge leap into his arms, then trust he would catch us, only to be catapulted high in the air and land gracefully on the other side. I nailed it every time. Each time I got higher and higher, and there was no doubt, Confidence and Strength, you were beneath my wings that day.

All of this to say, everything I learned from you both in all of my dancing days translated into my life. I took the leap on what felt worth taking a chance on, I learned how to pivot and change weight and directions when things didn't feel aligned. I kept my head up and eyes on my spot of focus when spinning out into the dark unknown, and today, whenever things feel like neither of you are nearby, I still put the music on and remember that I am fierce and just keep on dancing.

Thank you for your presence over the years. You built me into my force of nature which I am sincerely grateful for.

With love,

Phoebe

Where to Find Authentic Confidence

Strength and Confidence are two gifts that I believe rely somewhat on the balance of the external world, in how it both challenges you and nurtures you. I do feel you can invoke it within yourself but if they do not come naturally there needs to be some inner work first on clearing it up. Maybe that means first looking at some of the shadows of fear, shame, guilt, or resentment before you can truly hone in on your authenticity of Strength and Confidence.

I think these two are easy to mask to a certain extent. Strength, I feel you can fake it until you make it and that is actually what needs to happen to believe you have it. You may never know what you are fully capable of in terms of how strong you will be. That is up to life to decide based on the challenges it throws at you and how you respond.

Now if you lack Confidence at your core, and hide your insecurities, you can come off as cocky, egotistical, or even narcissistic. Playing with Confidence requires a lot of inquiry to truly know if it is authentic. It is not just about celebrating your wins but also reflecting in a healthy way those moments of failure and challenge. If you can be humble in sharing who you are authentically you will embody Confidence and Strength at your core.

Radiantly Confident in the Solar Plexus

In our subtle energy body, we look to our solar plexus where the fire resides to get us to take action, to build our strength, and to move willfully forward with confidence. When I think of Confidence, I think of being lit up from the inside. I feel it in my gut when I know something is meant for me. What about you, where do you feel it in your body when you just know something is meant to be for you? There might be a little bit of shakiness but when Confidence is present, it usually feels grounded, powerful, centered in the truth, a "meant-to-be-ness" right in the core of your being.

When we don't feel confident, or perhaps even feel some kind of resistance, things may feel off and not *right* at our core. That's when we tend to not feel confident about taking the next step forward when these feelings come up. There might be hesitation to take action because we fear our safety or question if it is aligned with our truth.

Both feelings, Confidence and Strength, come from our center, where we take action. Think about when we must physically move with power and strength, we have to move our legs to get us from point A to B. This is the action of a deep hip flexor muscle, the psoas. We even sometimes call this the fight or flight muscle that gets our legs to run and take immediate action. If we don't feel aligned with an action energetically, if we are not feeling confident, we may feel off in this area. I remember when I was hesitant about going through the next steps in my young adulthood: my dance career, and my marriage. I had a deep sensation that felt like a pain in my psoas that spoke to me pretty loudly until I felt confident about my choice in the next steps forward in my life. Once I made my choices, the noise quieted down, and I felt more aligned again.

Our diaphragm is also in the center of our body, our solar plexus, where we take deep breaths to cool ourselves down when there is too much fire, too much intensity, or too much action. We slow down our breath, we get quiet, and connect back with our center to listen to what the body needs to stabilize. So, at our center, we also know that action is not always necessary to keep the fire of our being going, sometimes it is a breath or a breeze to keep it steady.

There is more evidence today about how balancing the gut biome is the key to keeping the body strong and healthy. I have even read studies saying that keeping our emotional body healthy is also the key to keeping our gut-brain healthy since it is so sensitive to emotions like anger, anxiety, and sadness. It is important to note, we can't eliminate these emotions (I truly hope you figured that out by now with my overall message of this book), but if we are resilient and strong enough, we can take on anything that comes our way.

As you move through the next section, try to listen from your gut to what comes up.

Let's Check In

Here are a few questions you could ask yourself:

- Who was supportive in my life that helped me build Confidence?

- What experiences allowed me to shine my light?

- Who challenged me and did they do it in a healthy way?

- What experiences challenged me to be stronger and more resilient?

- Do I consider myself to be Confident? Why or why not?

- Do I consider myself to be Strong and Resilient? Why or why not?

Once you have a better gauge of where you are on the spectrum of healthy confidence and strength, invoke more of it into your life by exploring a few of these practices.

Power Songs. Before you have to press forward on something that is challenging or need to pump yourself up to make the next move, put on a power song that will pep you up, and if you feel so inclined, DANCE!

The higher the energy, the more positive you feel.

Sing it out, dance it out, know that you got this!

This was my go-to before auditions. I always had my playlist ready while I got on the train and powered my way through the busy city stress so that I would walk in and be ready to take on whatever count of eight they threw at me.

Power Outfits. One of my favorite pastimes as a kid, and

I still do it on occasion, is playing dress-up. Trying on a new look can feel empowering and maybe even get you to a place of believing a side of yourself you didn't know was possible. Make sure you are in good light and good headspace, then try on an outfit that makes you feel bold, sexy, confident, powerful, whatever you want to feel, and do your own catwalk. You own it! Even better, combine it with the power song and *get up offa that thing!*

Make an Awesome List. Write a list of all the ways you are awesome and how you love yourself. Feel free to add accomplishments (big and small), qualities you love, moments that challenged you and you overcame, and whatever else flows to celebrate you.

Protective Figure. If these practices were challenging, envision a supportive figure for yourself. This can be a real person who has always been there cheering you on, protecting you from harm, or it could be an archetype, a superhero, an angel, or whatever you want it to be. Then get really descriptive about this figure. What do they look like, smell like, sound like, what do they say to you to help you in challenging moments or help celebrate you? Meditate on these details for a little while and write in your journal all that you see in this protective figure. Then, ask how can you embody these qualities within you *for yourself?*

Now, whatever you are feeling in this moment, finish this statement:

As I step into my life with more Confidence and Strength, I embody the story of...

Letter to Love and Connection

Dear Love and Connection,

Why have I hesitated writing to you? Why does this feel like the hardest letter to write? Love, we humans talk about you, want you, admire you, long for you, will do anything for you, and share endless stories of finding you and losing you. You would think we would get you by now, myself included. I feel like you should be simple and easy, but we make you out to be so complex. What gives?

As I write this, I am not sure if it's right for me to say that I often get the two of you, Love and Connection, confused, do I mistake you for one another, or are you really the same thing? I feel like you should be the same thing, but I have more stories to say you are not. Let me see if I can explain myself instead of rambling.

Love, there are so many types of you, I can't keep track. Unconditional Love is the one that seems to be the simplest but so many people just don't believe in it. I do though; this version of you, I think I get. This is the love between myself and my parents that I was born with; it was in their eyes as my soul looked up for the first time and focused on their faces and they made "goo goo gaga" sounds at me. Of course, it got a bit more complicated the older I got, and I could feel their energy if it was not fully aligned with you. I think I can safely say, I never felt unloved by them. The moments I held onto when I saw my mom and dad cuddling together on a chair and I asked, "Can I join in?" reinforced that love. My request was never denied. I felt for the most part that I would always get a hug if I asked for it. For those darker moments with Dad, those days I felt abandoned by Mom, I felt alone and isolated but never not full of you, Love. It was more the lack of you, Connection.

When I was married, John and I used to contemplate the Unconditional version of you, Love. I believed in you, and I believed I had this for John. I still do, but he never believed you were real. It was our last conversation the day he stormed out, the day I knew there was no turning back. I still want the best for him and wish him Happiness and Love. Will you let him feel you, Love, if he hasn't yet? I was hurt by him, but never once did I stop loving or caring for him. I felt he couldn't believe in you because he was scared. He got in his own way because he lacked another version of you, Self Love. How can anyone believe they can be loved by someone if they don't love themselves first?

I also saw this, or the lack thereof, in my parents' reflections. When I was really young, I looked at Mom and Dad in the mirror. I was so very puzzled by what I saw there. They didn't look like "the real version" of themselves, their noses looked funny. I would ask them about what they saw and try to explain that I saw something much different. One time I looked at Dad's reflection when he was shaving and I thought to myself, "If he only knew what I saw, he would be amazed!"

For me, I think I have had a pretty good sense of the Self Love version of you, aside from when Shame and Guilt clouded my view of you. I also think my unconscious addiction to Chaos sometimes led to self-sabotage. In retrospect Love, had you been providing me with a solid foundation, those choices Chaos gave me would not have been on my radar as choices at all. It's okay though, I forgive us both. We still had fun or learned lessons in the end.

There are so many other ways of experiencing you, Love, through doing what I enjoy, nature, friendships, compassion and empathy for others, and romance. The Romance version of you we need to talk about, for myself and anyone else reading this. We need you to send out a press release or manual or something. Seriously, Love. Why is this one so hard to understand, feel, receive, and keep alive? You can watch any TV show, movie, read any book, or scroll on social media and at some point, you are going to bump up against this version of yourself. Why are we so obsessed with you in this form? Why can't we enjoy Self, Unconditional, Friends, and then stop right there? Why do we have to muck you up, get too attached, or be afraid of you? What gives? I want to solve this one for myself and all my friends out there. Why are you such a mystery if we don't have you? When we get you, you become too boring or tedious to keep the mystery alive. Romantic Love, what are my friends and I missing here?

My personal story with you is that I had a messed-up blueprint, I know this. I am the classic case of what they call the girl with Daddy issues. He was my emotionally unavailable knight in crappy armor that I constantly searched for in all my romantic relationships (notice past tense, please). I accepted anything I could get of you from men, who were maybe not the best fit for me. Well, perhaps not the best fit for me now, but they were exactly what I needed and wanted then. I still love all of them for who they were and what they taught me about myself and the world.

I do think my first young crushes were all good, sweet guys, but I broke up with them as soon as we got close, and they might find out about my home life. I was both embarrassed and protective of my situation.

My first real love was my high school beau. He was the one who drove us around drunk and high, and I sat in the passenger seat wide-eyed and ready for excitement in all the ways we explored together. He was a dark and twisty teen, perhaps a reflection of what I was not showing the world about myself at that time. What we felt you could not put into words; it wasn't tangible, but it was palpable, perhaps it was you, Connection. We had these intense feelings for each other and knew when the other person was thinking about the other. The physical distance wore on us over the years and looking back, there was the emotional distance too that I had not been aware of.

This emotional distance was the hallmark of all my romantic relationships after that until recently, simply because it was what I knew my whole life. I fell in love with great guys who just didn't know how to get out of their way. It was like they were carrying a backpack full of rocks while pushing a boulder up a mountain when all they had to do was let it all go and just walk. I thought and felt if I loved them so much it would make up for their lack of Self Love. This got really old. I am so done with this story with you, Romantic Love. I let go of my backpack full of rocks and stopped pushing the boulder up the mountain, and now I am just prancing around alone and trusting this version of you will come soon so I can have a playmate who can uplift me because he no longer has his unnecessary weight to carry. Can you make that happen soon, please?

Now, this brings me back to you, Connection. Is there some kind of misunderstanding here? Let me explain. When meeting new people, particularly someone attractive of the opposite sex, I immediately check in with you and Intuition quickly to see what we've got. After a few minutes into a conversation, I will get a confirmation from Intuition, she whispers, "Yes." Then you send a big electrical shock followed by goosebumps through my body, especially if our hands touch, we bump up against each other, or hug. I take this as a positive sign from you too. I will admit, I used to get these moments confused between you and Love. As things progress though if I continue reading your signs, everything feels like it is flowing, and then suddenly, they disappear, cords are cut, no more of you, I feel lost, confused, and I question all three of you, Love, Connection, and Intuition. I know I am not the only one here. There are dating apps that demonstrate this every day in smaller waves repeatedly by swiping right, a few decent texts, maybe a date, and then ghosted as if it never even happened.

What I have observed within, is the more I feel you after spending a lot of alone time, the more I feel grounded and less in need of searching for those outer versions of you, Connection, in people, places, or things. I feel steady and trust more in what you bring me now. Hmm, maybe I just cracked that code a little bit.

Now, Love and Connection, I know after all this you will respond by saying, "We are everything!" I know we are all each other's mirrors, so we are all connected in some way and the thread that runs through all of us is you, Love. I do conceptually understand this simplicity of you two. So maybe after all this, the question is how do we humans get out of our way, drop the backpacks and boulders, and just dance and embrace you both?

With a big hug,

Phoebe

Contemplating Love

The beautiful thing is there is probably no wrong way to experience Love and Connection if you are open to it. Even if you feel as if you lack Love and Connection in some aspects of your life, there are other ways you can experience it. For me, as you see, I am contemplating the whole romantic love thing. For you, it might be Self Love or Unconditional Love between a parent or sibling.

My hope is that you have some kind of reference point to work with where you can see a prototype of what you *don't* want, not as a place of judgment or expectation but more as a contrast. When we experience contrast, we see what feels off. When you can feel in your body that the connection feels good or when it feels off, then you will start to make more authentic connections more consistently.

A couple of questions you can ask yourself when contemplating Love and Connection:

- Am I forcing this connection because I am a people pleaser and I just want this person to like me or because I am scared to be alone?

- Am I avoiding this connection because I am afraid to get close to this person for some reason?

What I have found for myself is that the more I anchor in Self Love, the answers to these questions become clearer, and Intuition's voice cancels out the voices of Desperation or Fear. So, focus on yourself. I already know if you got this far you are in a very good place.

Connection at the Throat

The most obvious energetic connection here between Love and Connection is the heart chakra. But as I explained before, I felt it was necessary to start with Gratitude in the heart space. I feel like the throat chakra is sometimes where we "mess up" our communication with others if we are not clear with ourselves first.

The throat chakra is where we communicate, not only how we speak our truth to others but also how we receive the truth of others. If it is not clear on either end, we have miscommunication. If the pathways are clear we feel seen, heard, felt, and understood. When we feel this, we can also feel the acceptance and love from others.

I do believe we have lots of work to do in the heart to be able to communicate in a loving way, especially to ourselves. What I have found on the days that I don't love myself very much is that the thoughts I am thinking to myself and the words I am saying to myself are running on old thought patterns. Maybe you don't believe you are worthy of something fantastic to come to you or you feel that you deserve that crap sandwich that was handed to you. If we start with our words to shift the truth about ourselves and the other people we are struggling with, we might just make a big perspective switch.

I have always had a hard time working in groups where people were negative and toxic. I found their words woven into my vocabulary and how I saw my world. Not just in that work environment but in everything else too. When I was able to have an intimate conversation with myself to regain how I felt about the situation in an honest way, it encouraged me to speak my truth and every time I saw things change. There was deeper respect and love for myself when I didn't allow their negativity to infiltrate my way of being. I felt more grounded in being more of a light in the situation that desperately needed it. As a result, the environment shifted, or I was able to leave peacefully knowing I said what needed to be said from a space of love.

Let's Check In

Here are a few ways to accept yourself and infuse yourself with more love.

Start with how you see yourself.

Write a Letter to Your Body. This can be a difficult letter to write but such an expansive opportunity. I suggest writing this letter and revisiting it a few months later and writing a follow-up because your relationship with your body will continue to evolve. Take time to live it, celebrate, thank it, say you are sorry to it, that you were angry at it, or whatever you need to come to a place of acceptance.

- What were/are you afraid of, ashamed of, and/or disappointed in about your body?

- What is a story where it was not seen/heard/respected?

- What were/are you grateful for, confident of, regarding how it came through for you?

- What is a story about how it was celebrated?

- Consider what else was happening in your life during these moments and how they were mirrored into your body.

A Loving and Nurturing Figure

- **Create a vision of someone** who embodies unconditional love for you. This can be someone you know personally, a character in a movie, or an archetype. You decide how you want to create this person.

- **Get really descriptive.** Write, draw, and create a vision board of what they look like. What kind of clothes do they wear, what does their voice and laugh sound like, what do they smell like, what do they enjoy doing/being?

- **Then explore how they make you feel.** What kinds of things do they say to you, how do they nurture you, and how does it feel when they do, and how do you respond?

- **Now, how can you embody this for yourself?** If this kind of love is what you need, don't wait around for her/him/them to show up. You become your best nurturer.

- **Repeat with any other love figure you want to invoke.** Romance, friendship, familial, etc.

Tell Someone You Love Them

- You can start small here, tell someone who already knows you love them but send them a bit more than the "I love you" message. If you know your own love language, send them a message through that. (If you don't, that is a whole other book. Just listen to how you like to communicate and/or receive love intuitively and move from there.) For me, I share my love through my words of acknowledgment, and I also am quite affectionate when I feel safe with the person.

- Share an unexpected love for someone. This could be a friend you don't know so well but admire or someone you watch from afar on social media. Acknowledge them in a way that feels safe and good for you. The other day, I met a dear friend with whom I connect every few months. We inspire and admire each other from afar. After one of our meetings, we hugged and he said, "I love you." It felt so warm to receive these words from someone I respect so much. You don't know whose day you will make by passing along a friendly gesture of love.

- Make amends or at least a time out with someone you are miscommunicating with. This is a hard one, I know. Think of someone you haven't spoken to for a while. Maybe there was a falling out that is still gnawing at you, or maybe your relationship is in that place right now. Send a neutral message, even just a friendly text saying, "I still love and care about you and we will get through this." The most important thing is that there is no expectation on your end. If you can send the love for the sake of loving that person, there can be subtle or very profound healing for you both. If it feels like there will be an expectation for them to reciprocate, your heart isn't in the right place, and it is best to hold off. I have done this a few times with people who are very dear to me and sometimes it felt good and other times, I still felt conflicted, but only when I didn't have a clear intention. Just ask yourself, "Is this a necessary step?" If it doesn't feel right, then perhaps send them a message energetically through a letter never sent or a prayer or meditation for them.

If you are not sure who to start with, sit in this meditation and see who comes to mind and commit to communicating your love for them.

Loving Kindness Meditation

This is a Buddhist meditation, also known as *metta*, that is a useful practice to remember we are all connected. Practice when you feel disconnected from someone or the collective in some way.

May I be safe, protected, and free from inner and outer harm.

May I be happy and content.

May I be healthy and whole.

May I experience ease of wellbeing.

Bring someone you love to your mind, bring them down to your heart, imagine he/she is sitting in front of you and say...

May you be safe, protected, and free from inner and outer harm.

May you be happy and content.

May you be healthy and whole.

May you experience ease of wellbeing.

Bring someone neutral to you (like a local barista you see every day) to your mind, bring them down to your heart, imagine he/she is sitting in front of you, and say...

May you be safe, protected, and free from inner and outer harm.

May you be happy and content.

May you be healthy and whole.

May you experience ease of wellbeing.

Bring someone that you have a difficult relationship with to your mind, bring them down to your heart, imagine he/she is sitting in front of you, and say...

May you be safe, protected, and free from inner and outer harm.

May you be happy and content.

May you be healthy and whole.

May you experience ease of wellbeing.

Bring all beings in this vast universe to your heart and say...

May all beings be safe, protected, and free from inner and outer harm.

May all beings be happy and content.

May all beings be healthy and whole.

May all beings experience ease of wellbeing.

Now, whatever you are feeling in this moment, finish this statement:

As I step into my life with more Love and Connection, I embody the story of...

Letter to Peace and Serenity

Dear Peace and Serenity,

I often felt you close as I drifted off to sleep as a very young girl when Mom would read to me at bedtime and rub my back. I felt myself float into your gentle arms and when Mom slowed down her words and her little rubs because she thought I was in your full embrace (but not just yet!), I would open an eye and request her to keep reading or ask her to rub my back "like this." I would show her by rubbing my little fingers on her arm to direct her in the right direction to meet you Peace and Serenity at the edge of my dreams.

The nights Gramma came to visit, or I visited her, I also felt your presence, particularly when she told me my favorite story, "One Eye, Two Eyes, and Three Eyes." I never quite made it past the song sung by Two Eyes to her sister, Three Eyes, to make her fall asleep. I held on to you as long as I could as I drifted on a cloud of bliss with you both.

There were other quiet moments I felt your presence during my youth like the summer nights I would sit and watch the fireflies light up and go up. It was only later in life that I realized this was meditation. Everything changed for me though, the night I watched the fireflies go up with the quickly fading memories of my parents and me together. After that, I tried to find you both, Peace and Serenity, on my own as I lay alone in bed with so many thoughts and worries in my head. I imagined a big vacuum sucking all those thoughts and worries out so I could drift to sleep and feel you on my way there, if only for a few breaths.

You came to me less and less throughout my teens during all those bad years with Dad and my twenties when I went off to college and lived in the city. I got familiar glimpses of you though when I walked through city parks and sat on benches. I closed my eyes to block out the crazy world that was just beyond the tree-lined streets and feel the warmth of the sun on my face. When I found you both, it felt like distant friends that I just remembered, I had your number the whole time.

Then I found my way to the yoga mat. I dropped down into your gentle embrace again when I found savasana. It was like the physically challenging class stripped all the layers that kept me from feeling you, and there you were, holding me again. I remembered you, the fullness of you, and I craved you. I called on you more through my practices. Still living in a crazy world, I began to see you were a choice. Some days were harder than others, but I continuously showed up on my mat.

Then I got married on a really beautiful day. You two were with me to some extent, but I think it was really when we arrived in Grenada for our honeymoon that I fully felt your presence. While we sat watching the sunset eating delicious dark chocolate and drinking red wine, I felt you both so very deeply internally and externally, it all lined up. At that moment, you both sang in such harmony, not a key was off. I wondered if it could ever be possible again to experience this feeling of you. I had arrived in what felt like paradise, with a man I loved and was committed to, indulging in my favorite things, and everything was just "right." Ironically, this was probably the moment that shifted everything just ever so slightly to change the trajectory of my life. When I returned home, I decided to continue to make choices to invite you in more, not just on a yoga mat or on vacations. I wanted you both, Peace and Serenity to become my new life partners, which made my bed with my husband a bit crowded, I guess you could say.

I began to practice yoga more so I could understand you, receive you, and share your magic with others. I made new choices like spending more time with animals and in nature, to the point where we moved out of the city to be closer to you. I naturally found quieter moments with you while eating a meal, sitting with a furry friend, walking in a silent snowfall, or putting my feet in the Earth, and its waters. The closer I got with you, the further my husband and I drifted apart without fully seeing what was happening. He didn't know you as I knew you both and that may have threatened him in some way. Maybe he didn't trust you or feel safe with you, or maybe he still had the obstacles he needed to get through to be able to receive your honest embrace. It broke my heart when we parted because something inside of me felt he might not ever get to know you like I do, in the genuine, authentic ways that we know each other. He masked it and pretended to know you, but it was our friend, Numbness that he invoked to get a quick fix of what he thought was the two of you. That is his story now.

I walk my path with you both as my guides. I will admit, sometimes you offer me directions and it takes me a bit of time to follow. Sometimes, I stubbornly go another way down a long, winding, chaotic road, but I do find my way back to you, Peace and Serenity. I know now how to find you again, three deep breaths are my call to you, and then there you are. It may take a bit longer to surrender to your embrace again, but you are there, you are always there just waiting patiently for me.

You are here now in the butterflies that are curiously stopping by at the edge of my journal as I write these words. You are in the bird songs that came from the trees in my yard just a moment ago. You are in my shoulders as they soften away from my ears, I hear you whisper "relax," and in my feet and legs as they anchor in the ground and chair that I am sitting on. You are everywhere.

Even as I look up and see big, dark clouds rolling in, I feel your presence because you, Peace, are giving me a little respite from the hot sun and if these clouds should pour their waters down upon me, I know that Serenity is just beyond them with a cool breeze. Thank you for always being here, within me and around me. I bow to your grace and love.

With tenderness,

Phoebe

The Inner Journey of Serenity

How do you experience Peace and Serenity?

Are there moments you remember you felt their loving embrace and could not help but surrender to them?

Think about this for a moment: Did you ever experience the two just externally? I didn't think so. Peace and Serenity must be felt internally. Sure, we can use external factors to set the stage for us to receive the warm, fuzzy, calm feelings within, but we can't go searching for it outside of ourselves. If you don't have a close relationship with these two angelic friends, your whole external world could be completely serene, but you still might not be able to get "there" unless you go deep within yourself. But the beautiful thing about these two friends is that the world could be completely spinning out of control, yet if they are within you, that outer noise has nothing on you.

Something also to consider is our parasympathetic nervous system (PNS). Remember, this is your rest and digest system when things start to calm in the body, and you return to more of homeostasis. When your nervous system can switch over from the sympathetic nervous system (fight, flight, or freeze) to the PNS, you will get closer to this feeling of Peace and Serenity naturally. Invite practices like yoga, meditation, gentle movement, or anything that brings you joy to initiate the shift and then keep surrendering to their warm embrace.

Third Eye on Peace

This is the space above our eyebrows, where our third eye resides. The eye that sees inward, listens to our inner voice, our intuition. This is a voice that knows our truth and guides us to a place of expansion, deep knowing, and sensing. The more we can tap into Peace and Serenity, the closer we come to deep listening and seeing. As I shared in my letter, the outer noise and inner mind chatter get quieter when we connect with Peace and Serenity. We begin to see that there is so much in this outer world that is unnecessary, the man-made suffering, and that we have a choice in how we dance with it or leave it be. This is something we need to tap more into for ourselves, this third eye space, if we want to continue on with humanity.

We have to begin to see more clearly, listen to our inner voice and each other with clear intentions of love. When the voices that we call *vrittis* in Sanskrit (the fluctuations of the mind) get in the way, we don't see clearly, we don't think clearly, we don't hear clearly which often spiral us into the shadows of doubt, fear, anxiety, and judgment. Finding practices that resonate with you and allow you to clear out the clutter of the mind-stuff will allow you to drop down into trusting your inner voice. What I feel is necessary to emphasize is that you don't have to be a yogi, an expert meditator, or pray to a higher being or deity that you may or may not believe in to get to Peace and Serenity. It has to be authentic; it has to feel aligned with you and your natural state of being. If you like to be around animals, do that. If you like to be in nature, do that. If you like to be alone and draw, do that. Do what *feels* good so that the chatter gets quiet, and listen again to the inner voice that wants to play with you, wants to thrive with you, wants to protect you, and wants you to be happy.

What this inner voice should *not* sound like is someone outside of yourself telling you who you should be or what you should be doing. It doesn't judge you. It doesn't tell you that you have to be a certain way or do a certain thing that may cause harm to yourself, others, other creatures, or our planet. Our inner voice knows that we are all connected and works from this deep knowing because if you hurt yourself or something or someone else, you hurt us all. Our inner voice sees the bigger picture of the collective and our little being belongs in the vast, ever-expanding Universe. It sees it all and knows you belong. It knows you need to find Peace and Serenity in that knowing and will help you if you let it. So, get quiet and listen.

Let's Check In

Take a little bit of time to reflect on how Peace and Serenity feel for you.

Your Place of Serenity

Do you have a safe place or a happy place you can recall to set the tone? (If not, you can make it up. Imagination is a great place to start.)

What external factors invite Peace and Serenity closer to you?

- The scent of lavender?
- A deep meditation?
- Sitting by water?
- A calming song?
- The feeling of your feet in the sand?

What qualities does your body experience as a result? Some examples might be...

- Do your shoulders relax?
- Does your breath slow down?
- Does your mind pause from the monkey mind?

Write in your journal for five to ten minutes.

You can also use this as a way to meditate/visualize when you feel yourself being pulled into a stressful state of doing to shift back into a state of being.

What you want to make sure of is that this practice is not a way to escape, but to truly infuse the essence into your present moment.

Can't get there from here?

Get Your Ya-Yas Out

If you feel really wired up, try moving the body to a place of exhaustion. My teacher, Jeanmarie, would call this "getting your ya-yas out."

Maybe that means you have to put on a song that will make you move around to sweat or express a shadow feeling that has been repressed for some reason. Allow yourself to feel fully and then, once you are at a point of exhaustion, rest and receive the gift of Peace and Serenity.

Turn it All Off

Turn it all off. Turn off social media, media, TV, phone, people who spout negative chatter. Turn it all off for just a day and see how you feel. Then do it for two days, and then perhaps longer. Do something you love, see what voice reappears, maybe it is that long-lost friend, Intuition, who you can reconnect with again. Start to make choices from *this* place.

Need a little help at night?

Turn Your Brain Vacuum On

One of my favorite things to do as a child was another visualization I have mentioned before.

I would lie in bed and think of all the things I could possibly think about, let them crowd up my head. Then, I would imagine a big vacuum at the back of my head in my pillow; I would flip the switch and watch all the thoughts get sucked out until I drifted into a deep, peaceful rest. Try it!

A little extra help is to lie with your legs elevated. Slide them up a wall, place them on an ottoman, or even on a few pillows. This slight inversion will also calm the nervous system.

Now, whatever you are feeling in this moment, finish this statement:

As I release the tension and allow Peace and Serenity to infuse me deeply, I embody the story of...

Letter to Joy and Happiness

Dear Joy and Happiness,

Recently I heard about a billboard advertisement for a very popular online store that said, "Happiness is just one click away." I immediately threw up in my mouth a little bit. That's what most people believe, or rather have been conditioned to believe, about the two of you. Luckily, my mom ingrained in me at an early age that "Joy was found in experiences, not things." Sure, I was a lucky kid that got presents under my tree at Christmas. There is even a photo or two of me with my mouth gaped wide open as I entered our living room on Christmas morning to find out how lucky I was with Santa.

My parents were not rich. When I was a baby, we lived off welfare for a bit, and after they split up it was even more evident how we were lower middle class. But I was always grateful for what we had and what was given to me. What filled me up with the two of you most during the Christmases after my parents split were the letters my mom wrote me for Christmas when we were not together. I still have them. She usually wrote about the story of my first Christmas as a baby at the cabin and when my eyes lit up looking at the Christmas tree lights. The letter always ended with what my Christmas gift would be that year.

I remember I had to spend one Christmas with my dad in South Carolina at my grandparents 'house. There were presents under the tree for me that I had unwrapped early that morning but what I jumped up and down for was my annual letter from Mom. I was alone in my room and read that she registered me for classes at a prestigious ballet school in my area. I ran out to my dad to tell him the news, I was leaping and dancing around full of the two of you, I could not contain myself! I remember seeing my grandparents looking at me puzzled that I was not this joyful about the sweaters they got me.

I am grateful to have felt the truth of you both in these moments, and not lost in the things.

When I was young, I was filled with you both so often that I probably didn't recognize when you were there; I noticed you Joy and Happiness more when you were not there.

You were in my dance moves whether with friends or alone, performing, rehearsing, or just having fun. You were in me as I played with my friends at sleepovers, spent time with Gabby riding bikes, exploring together in our neighborhood, or just being silly with her brothers. You were in the laughter and tears I brought to my mom, my aunts, and my gramma when I made them play dress-up with me or made them laugh with my very strange "Pinky" voice. You were there on those summer nights I played outside and danced around with the fairies and fireflies that I sometimes caught in a jar for brief moments because I knew their Joy and Happiness were experienced in their freedom of flight and light.

When I got a bit older, you two came to me through dance opportunities accompanied by Enthusiasm, Inspiration, Gratitude, and Appreciation. I shared you both during slow dances with crushes, kisses, and phone calls with my boyfriends.

When I went off to college, I felt a bit distant from you because I was surrounded by artists who thought it was cooler to be dark and twisted by complaining about life and getting drunk to have a false sense of feeling for you both. I had glimpses of you in my twenties but remember struggling to get you close. There was a brief period when I made up a happy dance which was something I had to do when I was feeling down. John and I made it into a game we both played. If one of us was feeling shitty, we had to do it until we were smiling and laughing, and it usually worked.

The year I got engaged and when I was married, you both were so very present along with Love and Connection. Nothing really could have gotten between us during that year, Joy and Happiness. I was absolutely glowing.

You were there in my reunion with my dad, in that first hug we shared after eighteen years since the last time I saw him when he shoved me out the door on that rainy night. All the years we both missed you, and then we felt you again in that first hug and all the other hugs we got to share in the following four years. You both stayed close by while we reconnected. After he died though, it took some time to allow you back in. I felt you more on a subtle level within my grieving as I received mystical messages from him to keep going. Since then, I have begun to feel your presence more and more authentically from within, despite the external factors.

In 2019, my mantra was to "Move with Joy." I gave up my apartment to be more nomadic so I could really make choices that were aligned with you both, Joy and Happiness, not from stress, money, or fear. When I intentionally aligned with you both, I began to feel how everything was infused with you. By the time 2020 came around, I felt a great sense of freedom and shifted my word to "Trust" to be grounded in knowing that you two were always present in the process of my life unfolding. When the threat of the lockdown was approaching, I was in Bali. Although I was somewhat lost and confused, like all of us were that March, I knew you would guide me to a safe place that would allow me the deepest experience of you both. And I was right.

I arrived in West Virginia to be with my family, had the freedom to go inward, and build a stronger relationship with you both, which was such a gift. While the world was being tossed around in chaos, I watched in awe as a baby fox played in our yard. I danced in my room like I was young again, I wrote this book, I healed my mother wounds as I listened to stories about my gramma's childhood and contemplated different realms of reality with my mom. I would check back in with the outer world and see that they were still in the sea of chaos, anxiety, anger, separation, isolation, confusion, and grief. I'd shake my head in disbelief that my human friends still don't get you, Joy and Happiness. So, I sit here now and wonder how we can let you both be seen, heard, and felt across our world and Universe to shift our consciousness. I know the three of us can't do it alone. So, my dear friends, Joy and Happiness, how can we recruit more people? Maybe this story is one way to get them closer to you. Tell me, show me. I will continue to play, dance, and sing out of gratitude for you in hopes that others will hear and join in. I am doing my small part for all of us, and I am humbled you somehow chose me to be one of your ambassadors.

with light and love,

Phoebe

Our Duty to be Joyful and Happy

When are we going to realize that Joy and Happiness are our divine purpose, and it is what is humming underneath it all? Think about how much more fun life would be!

What if we allowed ourselves time to wander, roam, dance, play, and feel free again until the fireflies called us back home?

After I chose to move with Joy, I started to also change the way I moved in relationship with my physical, mental, emotional, and spiritual practices. I had been so very disciplined that it had become joyless. So, I made a conscious choice to let loose a little bit and create Unstructured Time for Play. What I discovered was that I was still practicing but less formally and there were subtle changes in how I was choosing to move and feel while doing them, as you will learn more below. Letting go of the expectations of what I felt like I was supposed to do and feel, opened a whole world of possibilities I didn't even know existed. In some of those times, I ended up developing my own movement practice Mvt109™ and writing this book!

A Crown of Joy

This is our final destination in the subtle body of our chakras. The crown chakra is how we connect to what is beyond. It is an open channel for communication with the divine, and you can call it God, Goddess, Universe, Fred, whatever you want. I believe it works with Intuition to remind us that everything is connected.

What does this have to do with Joy? The deeper I go into my life experiences and studies, I am convinced that Joy is humming underneath everything, and it is a choice. It is humming underneath grief, suffering, anger, numbness, all of it. It might be a little deeper under the surface at times for you to recognize it, feel it, or see it, but it is there, waiting patiently for you and ready with a big, sunshine-filled embrace! It is those moments we least expect that catch us in awe of life, from a baby's smile when we are having a wretched day, to the cute kitty that is asking to be petted, to when we are crying our own eyes out from our last break up, to a hug from a friend we bump into that we haven't seen in years as we rush to the train station. It is always here, ready to be seen, heard, and felt.

Our crown chakra is the gateway to our Joy. I like to think of our crown as our personal dot, our connection, to all the other dots in the matrix where we all live together in this Universe. When we go off our path away from Joy, our crown sends out the message to the Universe, this matrix, to show us a reason to get us back on the path with Joy. This could be a bunny hopping outside your window or a cute puppy that wants to jump on you and say hello. Our Universe brings us an opportunity to feel Joy again, even if it is just a fleeting moment to remind us that it *is all fleeting*, and the choice is ours in how we experience it.

If there is anything you take away from this book, I hope it is this: Despite all the heartaches, traumas, obstacles, and challenging circumstances you endure in life, you always have a choice. In my own story, I sometimes ignored the divine's guidance to choose Joy, and other times I could not help but surrender to it. Even at the depths of my rock bottom, I was always able to see some kind of possibility, some light beyond, guiding me back. I hope this book is some guiding light from beyond to welcome you back into yourself again and to feel the Joy of being you, fully.

Someone wrote me a message today. Someone I have never met but who observes me through social media. He said that he didn't know how I did it. He called me "cheerfulness on steroids" and questioned how I can be so positive while holding space for others. Well, if you have gotten this far, you know that I am not always so cheerful. I also don't think that what I put out into the world, specifically social media, is inauthentic. I am truly grateful for my life, and I choose to express that and the joy I have for living whenever I can to inspire others to know we all have a choice.

I have made a promise to myself to always show what feels necessary to people. I share only what feels necessary to be of service to you or anyone else in that time and space. When there are moments I need to be vulnerable, I share them. When I want to celebrate, I may share that too. Yet, there is still so much to me that you will never see simply because I want to keep parts of me close for myself and those I am most intimate with. Why I say this is because my hope is you can see some kind of balance as we speak of Joy. Joy is not to disregard the pain, to put on a "happy" face, and just suck it up. Trust me, I did that, and I crashed. You probably have too and know this is not sustainable.

Choosing to live in joy is courageous. You have to look into the eyes of Anger, Grief, Fear, Depression and say, "I know who you are, and you can't take a hold of me as you did before! I choose Joy!" because once those waves of the shadows roll through you, Joy will be there ready to dance, laugh, and play.

Let's Check In

What I have found is that when I lean into time and spaces that are more joyful and aligned with who I am, the more I can infuse Joy into everything I do. Let's infuse more joy into your life. This is the practice I spoke of a little earlier about allowing Joy to be more spontaneous.

Start by asking some questions.

Do you want to make a new recipe, write a book, start a podcast, create new artwork, design a new app, or try something you haven't even imagined yet? I invite you into the space of possibility to do, or rather to be, just that. *Sounds good, right?* So how do you get there?

Unstructured Playtime for Joy

What is it? Time and space where you show up with the simple intention of experiencing Joy with no other expectations.

What happens there? Anything you want.

I am writing from this space right now. It began today with reading a book on the Akashic Field, which somehow brought me to a recent loss of a friendship that spiraled me into tears and feeling sorry for myself, which then led me to move my body and recognize a pattern that was holding on to grief and abandonment, to then drinking a yogi tea with the message:

"Life is best lived by focusing on your goals & dancing through all the other distractions." -Yogi Tea

I followed that message by dancing to musicals which brought me back to Joy. I remembered my intention to choose Joy even through the tears because the suffering came from joyful moments shared with someone and my attachment to what no longer is. That brought me to lie on my belly on the floor writing these words for you.

Joy is a choice. However, in the lands of meetings, spreadsheets, to-do lists, obligations, and social engagements, we can sometimes forget. Setting aside these times and spaces of Unstructured Playtime for Joy has brought me peace. I am giddy with excitement to share with you that there is a time/space right here, right now that you can play in and create with. You just have to choose it.

So how do you do begin to claim Unstructured Playtime for Joy? With these four simple steps.

- **Schedule your unstructured playtime.** Start with five to ten minutes and build up to one hour throughout your day. Schedule it on your calendar. Claim it. No one else will do this for you.

- **Create or find a space with no distractions.** Find places you can go to or create that will keep you away from distractions during your playtime. These can be quiet spaces where you will not be disturbed in your home (maybe even a closet!) or outside, if need be, and away from technology as best as you can.

- **Make a list of joyful possibilities.** Write in your journal a list of all the things you love to do/be that perhaps you think you don't have time for (i.e., writing, being in nature, dancing, baking, painting, etc.). Think of these as toys for playtime.

- **Show up and PLAY.** Arrive at your scheduled time and see what happens. Then, PLAY! What's *PLAY* you ask?

Try this:

Pause what you are doing.

Listen to what is here for you now.

Activate and bring awareness to how you want to feel at the end of your unstructured time.

Yes, say a full body, "Hell YES!" and give what it is you want to feel the expression. This can be through dancing, singing, writing, meditating, running, swimming in a lake, whatever you want! Just go PLAY and move with JOY!!!

Now, whatever you are feeling in this moment, finish this statement:

With Joy and Happiness within me, I embody the story of...

FINALE

Please send me your last pair of shoes,
worn out with dancing as you mentioned in your letter,
so that I might have something to press against my heart.

— *Johann Wolfgang von Goethe*

A Final Letter to You

Dear Radiant One,

What a journey we have been on together! We are coming to the end of this part of our path. What's it been like for you? Through my story of shadows and light, how was your life reflected?

What did you learn?

What did you let go of, transform, or create for yourself from this experience?

Where were you resistant or expansive?

How did my words resonate with you?

Did it feel like coming home in some way, like remembering that you are a powerful creator of your own life and can make choices to embody and empower you in how you see, shape, experience, or feel it for yourself and the rest of our world?

I want you to know this process for me has been grueling. I had many moments when I paused and asked myself why??!?! Why am I doing this to myself? Why am I being called to share so much of myself, my intimate moments that have only been between me and pages in my journals hidden in my closets for most of my life? The vulnerability I feel is quite thick and I tremble a bit when I think about the actuality of you and anyone else out there reading it, but at my core, I am calm because I know in my bones it is all true and necessary to share.

Whenever I do anything that feels like it might be of importance and I am not sure if it is coming from ego or soul, I get quiet and ask within, "Is it necessary?" and then I listen. If it is a simple word, then it is my soul speaking, if it goes all crazy with rambling, it is ego. I invite you to ask this question while on your path and see what comes up for you.

So, there is one more story to share before we say goodbye. Before I do, I feel the call to highlight something first. The journey I shared with you was all done on my own. What I mean by this is I had teachers, therapists, guides, family, friends, books, practices, to support me and I am forever grateful for them all, but I was never reliant on one person like a guru or things like a pill to pop or plant medicine. This all came from very deep listening to life's call to awaken within so that I could better serve you and anyone else I may touch. I share this because the final story here did lead me to better understand myself and our world, but it was orchestrated by the Universe in its divine way. I did not search it out to think it would heal me and in fact, it took me several months to feel grounded and safe again. As you may already know, I am a rather sensitive human being. I say this because I am weary of the overuse and even somewhat abuse of plant medicine that is happening in the western world as a way to "fix" ourselves. It can be used as a tool that is meant to wake you up and then for you to continue your work and journey with other healthy resources, not to keep going back over and over to fix you. That is your responsibility, not anything outside of yourself.

This book took work for me and if you made it this far, I know it took a bit of work for you too, but hopefully with some lightness along the way. Now, let's come to the end...

It was the beginning of a new year, 2014, a year after my dad died and my marriage over. I ended up in Costa Rica for a reset. I thought I would only be there for a few weeks, but that day I had met a Tico who owned a restaurant in town, who helped me find a home and a job in one day so I could stay. That weekend was a music festival, Jungle Jam, the festival that I joked about coming back for when I was there a month earlier for a couple of days. I went with a friend I had met at the school I was attending for surf and Spanish. We saw my Tico friend there and he pointed us in the direction of the best food vendor who had ridiculously delicious empanadas. I also ran into another new friend, Branden who I learned shared a mutual friend back in the States which made me feel like he was a good person to connect and feel safe with.

We jumped into each other's arms and started dancing. There was an energy that felt different from other music festivals. Maybe it was the landscape with big prehistoric-looking trees towering over us along with palm trees and other tropical plants with flowers of every color imaginable. It was so different yet so comfortable and familiar. Maybe it was because I stayed at the hotel the month before and it already felt like home knowing I would be teaching there regularly in the coming weeks. Branden offered to share an edible weed cookie that he had just bought from a vendor. I hesitated.

I had always been extremely pensive about drug use because of Dad's abuse. I felt my body and mind were too sensitive to handle it. So, when Branden offered me a cookie, I hesitated but something told me to take it. I took a little bit and shared it with my other friend who was with me. We took a bite, then we all jumped into the crowd and started dancing. I felt so at one with everyone there dancing and feeling the music.

A bit later, I lost sight of my two friends and began to get nervous. I went to look for them. I got lost and tried to ground myself again. I went to the bar area to sit and take a breath. The energy of the music was too overwhelming. I found Branden and then everything he said I knew, like he was reading from some sort of script that I had written, or I had heard already several times. I looked at everyone and I felt that all the people around me were just playing their roles too; we all were. I didn't get it, but I did. I asked Branden to get me a bottle of water. I was feeling extremely weak and dehydrated. In my mind, I didn't like that part that was coming next. We stood in a large crowd to wait in some sort of line and then he was gone again.

I began to faint. Luckily, the people around me broke my fall and a classmate from the school caught me and brought me to a place away from everyone to sit. He was a cute Aussie from my Spanish class. We had only shared a few broken Spanish sentences in class over the previous two weeks. He sat with me to make sure I was okay. We started speaking like we had known each other for years, at least I did. I told him "I knew." He had no idea what I was referring to and gave me a puzzled look. I just kept saying, "I know, and it is okay. Your secret is safe with me." I had no idea what I knew either, but I felt guided to tell him that. He then broke down and said he didn't think anyone else could tell and he was grateful that someone else knew too. He held my hand a bit tighter in gratitude for seeing him. He was relieved and felt at peace with me knowing whatever his secret was.

From there, my entire world opened up as we sat together holding hands. It all made sense to me. I looked past the crowd of people at the festival and saw my entire life out around me, and others 'lives too, including Dad on the jungle floor after being shot down in Vietnam and experiencing a needle of heroin going into my veins as if I were him. It was like I was watching it all from a fishbowl but also living in it at the same time.

I relived all those moments of life again and again knowing I would circle back to sitting at the festival with this man who I barely knew by my side. I experienced the deep sadness of my new friend next to me and watched him display the faces of my past loves, Dad, and other men I had not yet met. He was all of them.

I desperately wanted to call Mom. I wanted her there with me to keep me calm. I kept looking at my phone to remind myself of time. Then, I raised my arms ever so slowly like a familiar dance and experienced the whole Universe within me. I saw all the lives within my movement, and I remembered how I had been here before when I was in my apartment in New York City, and even further back when I danced in my room as a child when I heard the word choreographer whispered to me from beyond. This was the Divine Contract that I had signed back then. I was the choreographer of my life, and within the entire Universe, I danced. I had entered back into perichoresis, encircled by a community of love in the flow of the Divine Dance.

It was truly the most peaceful thing I had ever experienced. But then my friend needed to go, and he left me there alone. It shifted me out of that divine moment of peace. There was darkness and much discord. My visions went back and forth between what was thought to be my past and what was thought to be the future. I was feeling the darker days of my past and the darker days ahead for all of us. It was hard to know where I was in the present, but I felt heartbroken like I lost my soul mate. It felt like an eternity waiting for him. Then, something pulled me out of it just as quickly as I fell into it. I heard a man's voice singing a gentle folk song and all these little white lights were surrounding me. It was all of our souls becoming free again. Each little white light paired up with another white light, which made them even brighter, and they flew up into the sky. Like fireflies, they lit up the dark sky and went up.

Fly on, Radiant One,
Fly On,

Phoebe

Acknowledgments

I would like to take a bit of time and space to express my deep gratitude for the people who helped me and inspired me along this journey.

My mom—For giving me the grace to share our story. Thank you for always loving me unconditionally and supporting me in all of your ways throughout my life. I have a feeling I don't even fully realize how much you have been there for me this whole time.

My dad—For being my most valuable teacher and guiding me through really hard lessons that have led me to wisdom that can only be accessed through experience.

Gabby—For giving me so many valuable memories that will continue to live on as I walk this earth with you in my heart.

My gramma—For being my own personal guru and for being so very beautiful (both inside and out) even if you don't fully see this in yourself. I treasure you.

My Aunt Betsy—For inspiring me to be an author.

My Grandpop Bob—For inspiring me to take the path as an artist.

For the rest of my family—For helping me share this part of my journey with ease.

My teachers (both in the classroom and in life):

> Jeanmarie Paolillo—For helping me change my vibration.

Elizabeth Andes Bell—For giving me the nudge to do things outside of my comfort zone.

Jillian Pransky—For giving support when I needed it the most.

Tao Porchon Lynch, Milton Myers, Bill T Jones, Shawn Cosby, Ila Gupta, Alexander John Shaia, Rob Bell, Elizabeth Gilbert and all the other teachers and healers for teaching and helping me heal on this path.

JK—For giving me the grace and strength to share these stories and all the wonderful and challenging years we shared and endured growing up together.

Michael—For being the first man who really saw me, looked into my eyes and said, "I'm sorry." That moment and our relationship taught me how to be truly vulnerable.

My other past loves for teaching me how to love and when to walk away still with love and admiration in our hearts.

Christy—For being my therapist during the most challenging time of my life.

My dear friends:

> Dante—For making me reverse it and on the left every time.

> Bri—For bringing my work to life with such integrity.

> Gisela—For bringing my love of words and movement together again and inspiring me to keep dancing.

> Pallavi, Meghan, Erika, Lori P, Amy S, Caryn, Paula and my other Hudson Valley community of friends for supporting me through this process.

TJ, Koko, Jeanmarie, Lori P, Amy G, Gisela, and Andrea for reading my words and reflecting back in a way that gave me clarity that this book matters.

My nOMad Community (past and present):

> Sam, Corinna, Juan-Carlos, Melia, Mike, Amy S, Amy G, Guru Bill, Koko, Jen E, Jessica, Lori, Emily, Erin, Nikki, Dani, Ally, Jen D, Jen P, Elizabeth C, Kadriya and all the Hudson Valley yoga studio owners, past trainees, and retreat participants for being a part of this beautiful community. nOMad could not have become what it is today without you!

Lea—For being a rockstar production manager, community manager, dancer, nOMad doula, nOMad teacher, Mvt109™ facilitator, mindful VA, and all things that you are and do for nOMad, Mvt109™, me, and our world.

The GracePoint Publishing team and Alexa of WEX for this life-changing opportunity.

Shauna—For being the person who read my words for the first time and allowed me to believe in myself and my voice.

Laurie—For your meticulous detail and optimism.

Tascha—For being such a calming presence throughout the whole process from the moment we met which gave me the trust and confidence to take this leap!

And finally, anyone who has believed in me for giving me the opportunity to be ME and share these stories and practices with our world to heal, grow, and expand.

Deep bow to you who reads this, Dear Radiant One...

About the Author

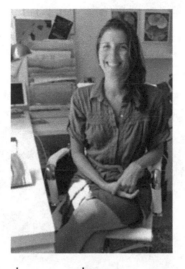

Phoebe Leona is a dancer, yoga teacher, and transformational guide who helps people feel more embodied through somatic, movement, and expanded awareness practices to become more empowered in who they are, who they are becoming, and have a greater sense of belonging. She has been a teacher and guide for most of her life but it was after a year of extreme loss in 2013 when she found herself in the vast open space in between her old life and a new life, that she dove deeply into her practices and began her company. nOMad helps others through their own transitions and the spaces in between. Throughout that time, Phoebe also developed her movement/somatic practice, Mvt109™ for students to fully embrace the freedom of moving in their bodies, transforming old and held patterns, and reclaiming the vibrations and stories they want to bring to life. Phoebe also finds joy in sharing her story to help others in their healing.

You can learn more about Phoebe's story on her TEDx Talk and her podcast The Space in Between.

For more great WEX Press books visit
Books.GracePointPublishing.com

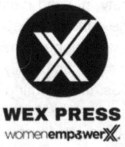

WEX PRESS
womenempowerX.

If you enjoyed reading *Dear Radiant One* and
purchased it through an online retailer, please return to the site
and write a review to help others find this book.